THE 22-DAY
REVOLUTION

ALSO BY MARCO BORGES

Power Moves: The 4 Motions to Transform Your Body for Life

THE 22-DAY
REVOLUTION

The Plant-Based Program
That Will **TRANSFORM** Your Body, **RESET** Your Habits,
and **CHANGE** Your Life

MARCO BORGES

WITH SANDRA BARK

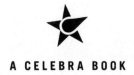

A CELEBRA BOOK

Celebra
Published by the Penguin Group
Penguin Group (USA) LLC, 375 Hudson Street,
New York, New York 10014

USA | Canada | UK | Ireland | Australia | New Zealand | India | South Africa | China
penguin.com
A Penguin Random House Company

First published by Celebra,
a division of Penguin Group (USA) LLC

First Printing, April 2015

Copyright © Marco Borges, 2015
Foreword copyright © Beyoncé Knowles Carter, 2015
Introduction copyright © Dr. Dean Ornish, 2015
Illustrations accompanying The 22-Day Revolution Exercise Routine and Power Foods:
    Nicole Hitchens
Photography for the Plant-Based Proteins chart: Ben Coppelman
Photo insert: Concept and photography by Ben Coppelman
Photography styling: Arlene Delgado and Ben Coppelman

THE LIBRARY OF CONGRESS HAS CATALOGED THE HARDCOVER EDITION OF THIS TITLE AS FOLLOWS:
Borges, Marco.
The 22 day revolution: the plant-based program that will transform your body, reset your habits, and change your life/Marco Borges with Sandra Bark.
p. cm.
ISBN 978-0-451-47484-1 (hardback)
1. Vegetarianism. 2. Diet. I. Bark, Sandra. II. Title. III. Title: The twenty-two day revolution.
TX392.B635 2015
641.5'636—dc23   2014043103

Printed in the United States of America
10 9 8 7 6 5 4 3

Set in Whitman
Designed by Pauline Neuwirth

I would like to dedicate this book to my wife, partner and best friend, Marilyn, for her constant love and support. And to my boys, Marco Jr., Mateo and Maximo, for being the Sun and the Moon in my life.

CONTENTS

PART THREE

GO!:
22 Days of Revolution Meal Plans

PART FOUR

POWER UP YOUR REVOLUTION:
Making the Program Work for You

PART FIVE

REVOLUTION FOR LIFE:
Recipes and Motivation for Day 23 and Beyond

FOREWORD

by BEYONCÉ

I WAS BORN AND RAISED in Houston, and if there's one thing we love in Texas, it's good food. Food has always been at the heart of my family, and it played a big role in my upbringing. We celebrated, bonded, commiserated, and loved one another through food—and not necessarily the healthy kind. Our hometown favorites were fried chicken, fajita tacos, BBQ burgers, BBQ ribs, fried shrimp, and po'boy sandwiches. Growing up, I was always on the move and didn't always make the right choices when it came to food and may have even developed some habits around it that were silently sabotaging my health as I grew older.

After having my daughter, I made a conscious effort to regain control of my health and my body. But I didn't want to do a crash diet. I was a mom now. I needed to change my ways and set an example for my child. So I turned to no one other than my good friend and fitness and nutrition confidant, Marco Borges. I've worked with him for years to keep me on-track, motivated, and ahead of the health game. Yet, as much as I follow and trust his advice, when I would hear him talk about the amazing benefits of a plant-based lifestyle, I would think, that sounds amazing. I would love to experience those benefits, and while I can incorporate those good foods into my life, I knew I could never eat that way. I love food too much. Something needed to happen for me to come around. I needed to be ready.

A year later (around November 2013), my husband and I decided we wanted to try a completely plant-based diet with Marco. I had lost my pregnancy weight with his help, through an exercise-and-nutrition program, and was ready for another challenge. I decided I wanted to take a more proactive role in my health, and knowing all the amazing benefits, I knew this was the one. I was ready.

And so the journey began that helped me get into the best shape of my life. Little did I know the long-lasting effects it would have. I thought, like with most diets, I would feel deprived and hate food, that I would miss out on restaurants and celebrations, that I would get headaches and be irritable, etc. I was wrong about all of that. It took a few days to adjust, but what I discovered was increased energy, better sleep, weight loss, improved digestion, clarity, and an incredibly positive feeling for my actions and the effects it would have on those around me and the environment. I couldn't believe how much of our health we can control with food. And that I *could* still love food but this time it would love me back (like the walnut tacos you'll find in here, oh my!!). We even celebrated my husband's birthday with an all-vegan party. I can still see the reaction on our friend's faces. Some were extremely excited while others had some reservations, but in the end, we all enjoyed it immensely. My greatest discovery was that I would benefit from the best gift I could give myself and my family—my health.

I'm sharing my experience because I want the best for everyone, and I would like for anyone who thinks that this isn't for them, even though they may know of the incredible benefits, that they *can* do it. You deserve to give yourself the best life you can. Empowerment starts within you and your decisions. You can control the quality of your life with the food you eat. The truth is that if a Houston-born foodie like me can do it, you can too—you just need to try it for 22 days.

—Beyoncé

INTRODUCTION

I WELCOME THIS OPPORTUNITY TO write the introduction to this important book, as awareness is the first step in healing.

For almost four decades, my colleagues and I at the nonprofit Preventive Medicine Research Institute and the University of California, San Francisco have conducted clinical research proving the many benefits of comprehensive lifestyle changes. These include:

- a whole-foods, plant-based diet (naturally low in fat and refined carbohydrates) like the one described in this book;
- stress-management techniques (including yoga and meditation);
- moderate exercise (such as walking); and
- social support and community (love and intimacy).

In short—eat well, move more, stress less, and love more.

Many people tend to think of advances in medicine as high-tech and expensive, such as a new drug, laser, or surgical procedure. We often have a hard time believing that something as simple as comprehensive lifestyle changes can make such a powerful difference in our lives—but they often do.

In our research, we've used high-tech, expensive, state-of-the-art scientific measures to prove the power of these simple, low-tech, and low-cost interventions. These randomized controlled trials and other studies have been published in the leading peer-reviewed medical and scientific journals.

In addition to *preventing* many chronic diseases, these comprehensive lifestyle changes can often *reverse* the progression of these illnesses.

We proved, for the first time, that lifestyle changes alone can reverse the progression of even severe coronary heart disease. There was even more reversal after five years than after one year and 2.5 times fewer cardiac events. We also found that these lifestyle changes can reverse type 2 diabetes and may slow, stop, or even reverse the progression of early-stage prostate cancer.

Changing lifestyle actually changes your genes—turning on genes that keep you healthy, and turning off genes that promote heart disease, prostate cancer, breast cancer, and diabetes—more than five hundred genes in only three months. People often say, "Oh, it's all in my genes. There's not much I can do about it." But there is. Knowing that changing lifestyle changes our genes is often very motivating—not to blame, but to empower. Our genes are a predisposition, but our genes are not our fate.

Our latest research found that these diet and lifestyle changes may even lengthen telomeres, the ends of your chromosomes that control aging. As your telomeres get longer, your life gets longer. This was the first controlled study showing that any intervention may begin to reverse aging on a cellular level by lengthening telomeres. And the more people adhered to these lifestyle recommendations, the longer their telomeres became.

This is a different approach to personalized medicine. It's not like there was one set of dietary recommendations for reversing heart disease, a different one for reversing diabetes, and yet another for changing your genes or lengthening your telomeres. In all of our studies, people were asked to consume a whole-foods, plant-based diet like the one described in this book. It's as though your body knows how to personalize the medicine it needs if you give it the right raw materials in your diet and lifestyle.

It's not all or nothing. In all of our studies, we found that the more people changed their diets and lifestyles, the more they improved and the better they felt—at any age. If you indulge yourself one day, eat healthier the next.

These lifestyle changes are part of the most influential trend in medicine today—what is known as "Lifestyle Medicine," which is lifestyle as *treatment* as well as prevention.

And what's good for you is good for our planet. To the degree we transition toward a whole-foods, plant-based diet, it not only makes a difference in our own lives; it also makes a difference in the lives of many others across the globe.

The crises in global warming, health-care costs, and energy resources can feel overwhelming: "What can I do as one person to make a difference?" This may lead to inaction, depression, and even nihilism.

However, when we realize that something as primal as what we choose to put in our mouths each day makes a difference in all three of these crises, it empowers us and imbues these choices with meaning. If it's meaningful, then it's sustainable—and *a meaningful life is a longer life.*

HEALTH CRISIS

More than 75 percent of the $2.8 trillion in annual U.S. health-care costs (mostly sick-care costs) are from chronic diseases that can often be prevented and even reversed by eating a plant-based diet at a fraction of the costs.

For example, in the European Prospective Investigation into Cancer and Nutrition (EPIC) study, patients who adhered to healthy dietary principles (low meat consumption and high intake of fruits, vegetables, and whole-grain bread), never smoked, were not overweight, and had at least thirty minutes a day of physical activity had a 78 percent lower overall risk of developing a chronic disease. This included a 93 percent reduced risk of diabetes, an 81 percent lower risk of heart attacks, a 50 percent reduction in risk of stroke, and a 36 percent overall reduction in risk of cancer, compared with participants without these healthy factors.

Another recent study of more than twenty thousand men found that those who didn't have much belly fat and who had a healthy diet, didn't smoke, and exercised moderately reduced their risk of a heart attack by 80 percent.

It's not just low-fat versus low-carb. A new study found that animal protein dramatically increases the risk of premature death independent of fat and carbs. In a study of more than six thousand people, those aged fifty to sixty-five who reported eating diets high in animal protein had a 75 percent increase in overall mortality, a 400 percent increase in cancer deaths, and a 500 percent increase in type 2 diabetes during the following eighteen years.

At the same time that the power of comprehensive lifestyle changes is becoming more well documented, the limitations of high-tech medicine are becoming clearer.

For example, randomized controlled trials have shown that angioplasties, stents, and coronary bypass surgery do not prolong life or prevent heart attacks in most stable patients. Only one out of forty-nine people with early-stage prostate cancer and PSA levels below ten may benefit from surgery or radiation. Also, type 2 diabetes and prediabetes are pandemic, affecting almost one half of Americans, yet drug treatments to lower blood sugar do not prevent the complications of diabetes nearly as well as lowering blood sugar with diet and lifestyle. United Health Care estimated that if current trends continue, the costs of type 2 diabetes will be $3.3 *trillion* by 2020, which is clearly not sustainable.

Lifestyle medicine is cost effective as well as medically effective. Our research has shown that when comprehensive lifestyle changes are offered as *treatment* (not just as prevention), significant cost savings occur in the first year because the biological mechanisms that control our health and well-being are so dynamic.

For example, Highmark Blue Cross Blue Shield found that overall health-care costs were reduced by 50 percent in the first year when people with heart disease or risk factors went through our lifestyle program in twenty-four hospitals and clinics in West Virginia, Pennsylvania, and Nebraska. In patients who spent more than $25,000 on health care in the prior year, costs were reduced 400 percent in the following year. In another study, Mutual of Omaha found that they saved $30,000 per patient in the first year in those who went through our lifestyle program.

Because of these findings, we are grateful that Medicare began covering our program of lifestyle medicine in 2010. If it's reimbursable, it's sustainable. (For more information, please go to www.ornish.com.)

GLOBAL-WARMING CRISIS

Many people are surprised to learn that animal agribusiness generates more greenhouse gases than all forms of transportation combined. The livestock sector generates more greenhouse gas emissions than the entire global transportation chain as measured in carbon dioxide equivalent (18 percent versus 13.5 percent). More recent estimates are that these numbers are even higher—that livestock and their by-products may actually account for more than 50 percent of annual worldwide greenhouse-gas emissions (at least 32.6 billion tons of carbon dioxide per year).

It is also responsible for 37 percent of all the human-induced methane, which is twenty-three times more toxic to the ozone layer than carbon dioxide, as well as generating 65 percent of the human-related nitrous oxide, which has 296 times the global-warming potential of carbon dioxide. Nitrous oxide and methane mostly come from manure, and fifty-six billion "food animals" produce a lot of manure each day.

Also, livestock now use 30 percent of the earth's entire land surface, mostly for permanent pasture but also including 33 percent of global arable land to produce feed for them. As forests are cleared to create new pastures for livestock, it is a major driver of deforestation: some 70 percent of forests in the Amazon have been turned over to grazing.

ENERGY CRISIS

More than half of U.S. grain and nearly 40 percent of world grain is being fed to livestock rather than being consumed directly by humans. In the United States, more than eight billion livestock are maintained; these livestock eat about seven times as much grain as is consumed directly by the entire U.S. population.

Producing one kg of fresh beef requires about thirteen kg of grain and thirty kg of forage. This much grain and forage requires a total of 43,000 liters of water.

So, to the degree we choose to eat a plant-based diet, we free up tremendous amounts of resources that can benefit many others as well as ourselves. I find this very meaningful. And when we can act more compassionately, it helps our hearts as well.

We're always making choices in our lives. If what we gain is more than what we give up, then it's sustainable. Because these underlying biological mechanisms are so dynamic, if you eat and live this way for just 22 days, you're likely to feel so much better, so quickly, you'll find that these are choices worth making—not from fear of dying but from joy of living.

For all these reasons and more, this is the right book at the right time. It can help transform your life for the better.

Marco Borges embodies the core values that he writes about in this book. What he describes here can make a powerful difference in your health and well-being.

The Harvard Health Professionals Study and the Harvard Nurses Health Study followed more than thirty-seven thousand men and eighty-three thousand women for almost three million person-years. They found that that consumption of both processed and unprocessed red meat is associated with an increased risk of premature mortality from all causes as well as from cardiovascular disease, cancer, and type 2 diabetes.

And it's not just the arteries in your heart that get clogged on a diet high in red meat. Erectile dysfunction—impotence—is *significantly higher* in meat eaters. In men forty to seventy, more than *half* report problems with erectile dysfunction.

Good news: according to the Massachusetts Male Aging Study, eating a diet rich in fruit, vegetables, whole grains and fish—with less red and processed meats and fewer refined grains—significantly decreased the likelihood of impotence.

It's not all or nothing. Start with a meatless Monday (or Tuesday or Wednesday). To the degree you move in this direction, there is a corresponding benefit.

You'll look better and feel better and have hotter sex and a cooler planet.

Now *that's* sustainable.

DEAN ORNISH, M.D.

Founder and President, Preventive Medicine Research Institute
Clinical Professor of Medicine, University of California, San Francisco
Author, *The Spectrum* and *Dr. Dean Ornish's Program for Reversing Heart Disease*
www.ornish.com

THE 22-DAY MANIFESTO

WE BELIEVE that success is a by-product of effort and consistency.

WE BELIEVE you should live the life you want,
not just the one you have.

WE BELIEVE we have the power to effect change.

WE BELIEVE in ourselves.

THE 22-DAY
REVOLUTION

PART ONE

CHANGE YOUR HABITS, CHANGE YOUR LIFE:

Why the 22-Day Revolution
Is So Effective

1

WELCOME TO THE 22-DAY REVOLUTION

IF YOU WANT TO CHANGE your health and make those changes permanent starting right this moment, you can. How? Begin by eating plants.[1] And by this I mean a whole-foods, plant-based diet with meals like walnut tacos, veggie ceviche, lentil soup, quiona-stuffed red peppers, oatmeal with banana and blueberries, chia puddia. So whenever you see "eat plants," I want you to think of delicious, live foods that make you look and feel amazing while inspiring the best in you.

Eating plants is the most powerful, most effective, and simplest way to get healthier. If you want to lose weight, if you want to be fitter and stronger than ever before, you must eat more plants. Obesity, heart disease, diabetes—all of these illnesses come from eating too much of the wrong kinds of food. If you regularly eat processed foods, from sugar-added cereals to meats that are pickled in preservatives, you are probably getting too many calories and not enough vitamins and minerals, and creating a situation where your body cannot help but gain weight and eventually become sick.

A plant-based diet will help you lose weight and keep it off; provide an enormous amount of energy daily; and prevent long-term health problems like heart disease and high blood pressure. A plant-based diet is the answer to some of the major problems plaguing our country, from

---

[1] When I say "right this moment," I mean it. Go eat a nice piece of fruit or slice up an avocado before you read another word. See, you've already started!

3

these increasingly commonplace diseases to the slow and steady break-down of the environment. "Eat plants" is a mantra that I live by, and one that I voice everywhere I go—to my family, friends, and clients—because I believe it to be the most important thing we can do to take care of ourselves and the planet that we live on.

I have learned firsthand during my twenty years of helping clients lose weight and regain health that diet is the most important tool that we have, and that a plant-based diet is the very best way to achieve vital-ity and longevity—and to get the best body of your life.

WHY IS PLANT-BASED EATING BETTER FOR YOU?

▶ **PLANTS HELP YOU LOSE WEIGHT.**
As your palate adjusts to the natural and whole foods you're eat-ing, cravings for processed and sugary foods subside.

▶ **PLANTS PUMP UP YOUR ENERGY.**
By eating an abundance of fresh fruits and vegetables, your body will be flooded with vitamins and minerals. And without expend-ing energy breaking down overprocessed foods, your body can focus on repair and cell renewal.

▶ **PLANTS INCREASE YOUR HEALTH FOR THE LONG TERM.**
As you'll find out in the coming chapters, a plant-based diet can help reverse heart disease, diabetes, hypertension, obesity, and other diseases that are caused by eating unhealthy, unwholesome, processed foods.

It may sound drastic, but a plant-based diet is actually one of the most common ways of eating. In fact, worldwide, an estimated four billion people live primarily on a plant-based diet, while only about two billion people live primarily on a meat-based diet.[2] Places where plant-based and vegetarian diets are most popular have far lower levels of health

---

[2] *The American Journal of Clinical Nutrition*, http://ajcn.nutrition.org/content/78/3/660S., accessed October 13, 2014.

problems, like high blood pressure and heart disease, than in Western countries. For example, India, a country that has the world's second-biggest population—more than 1.2 billion people!—has five hundred million vegetarians. What is radical is our Western style of eating meat, dairy, eggs, and processed foods. America's waistlines, health, and even the environment are paying the price.

Every time clients come to me with the desire—the need—to lose weight and regain control over their lives, I teach them how to incorporate more plants into their diets and cut out the over-processed foods that are slowly poisoning their bodies. With a true plant-based diet, I can help my clients drop anywhere from ten to one hundred pounds and radically transform their overall health. Within days and weeks, each one of them experiences firsthand the incredible benefits, like watching the pounds melt away while they catapult themselves into a world of energy and vitality, simultaneously reversing disease and improving their health profile.

The biggest obstacle I must first help them overcome is the idea that giving up meat and animal products is impossible. No bacon?! No cheese?! Yes. By giving up what you consider to be essential (and fun) components of your diet, you will gain so much more. Choosing plants regularly and discovering how delicious plant-based food is will create brain pathways that will support your newer, better habits. As you become more used to eating plants, and start to really feel the benefits, your new habits will become second nature, and it may soon become hard to imagine that you ever ate a different way.

The 22-Day Revolution program is a 22-day intensive program built to reset your body and mind. It will jump-start your body, so you can get healthy and shed the excess weight. It will be challenging, but as your body adjusts to the correct portions, you'll learn what 80 percent fullness should feel like. If you've been overeating for years, or are more than fifty pounds overweight, the portions outlined in the 22-day program will feel small. That's why the plan allows for healthy snacks as needed. If you're embarking on this program for its myriad health benefits instead of weight loss, then chances are the portions are much more in line with what you're currently consuming. This program is about change, creating new habits and breaking the ones that aren't working for you anymore. It's empowering to learn that you can completely transform the way you live and feel in such a short and manageable amount of time.

By combining the benefits of plant-based eating with breakthroughs in science about habit formation and development, I developed a program that, over 22 days, introduces people to eating plants, and simultaneously resets their habits in a way that makes plant-based eating more sustainable for the long term.

Many people begin healthy eating programs; not many manage to make those changes permanent. The goal of the 22-Day Revolution is to get you past the point where most diets fail so that you can create long-lasting change. When I was studying psychology, I discovered that some psychologists believe that it takes 21 days to make or break a habit. The human brain is an incredible machine that can rewire itself over time. The more often you engage in a specific behavior, the more pathways your brain builds to support that behavior. Scientists call that neuroplasticity: the ability of your brain to "change [its] connections and behavior in response to new information, sensory stimulation, development, damage, or dysfunction."[3]

Challenge yourself to introduce newer, healthier habits for 21 days, and on day 22, you will emerge as an improved version of yourself. If you can make it through three weeks, you can make it forever!

Gone will be the days of yo-yo dieting, the constant state of misery where you consistently rebound between eating too much, feeling too full, and gaining weight, to going on a strict diet and feeling miserable. Instead, you'll feel energized immediately, and over time the benefits will absolutely amaze you.

The 22-Day Revolution will give you the tools to take control of your life and your body, to learn to eat in a way that empowers you instead of slowing you down. Three weeks from now, you could be at the beginning of a brand-new way of living in the world—one that makes you feel happy and content.

And you are holding the map in your hand.

This program is a guide to losing weight and gaining health by learning to eat plants.

- It's a manual for habit change, so you can develop an awareness of the unconscious reactions that are ruining your health and making you gain weight.

---

[3] http://www.britannica.com/EBchecked/topic/410552/neuroplasticity, accessed August 18, 2014.

- It's 22 days of menus that will introduce you to fresh flavors while you learn new habits that will make you healthy and strong.
- It's a path of discovery, as you realize that it is possible to love food and lose weight at the same time, without guilt.
- It's an introduction to the true sensation of fullness, the optimal feeling after meals, which you can experience only when you learn to eat with restraint.
- It's a cookbook that will show you simply delicious and deliciously simple ways to prepare and enjoy all of nature's vibrant delights.

If you're looking for a way to lose weight, reclaim your health, and feel good about yourself through and through, it's possible. If you want to give yourself what you need to have an inner glow and an outer glow that inspires all of the people who know you to say, "What are you doing? Something about you is different!" you can. Food matters! And eating a plant-based diet will help you lose weight, feel better, and positively glow with good health. Plain and simple: It gets results.

Across the country, people are taking up the challenge: Spend 22 days on a plant-based diet and see what it will do for you. Are you ready to join us? If you're reading this book, I suspect that the answer is already yes.

Set your goals and create a road map for success. What are your personal goals? Do you want to lose weight? Do you want to change your health profile so that you'll be able to attend your child's graduation in fifteen years? Do you want to reverse heart disease, have more energy, encourage your family to be more healthful? Be mindful and clear about your goals, and consider writing them down so that you will have inspiration during hard days, and a reminder of what you set out to do so you can appreciate your progress as you move through the program.

In just 22 days you can change the way you feel about yourself, the way you feel about the world, the way you feel every single day.

A SIMPLE CHANGE, INCREDIBLE RESULTS

Every time a client takes the challenge, I get an e-mail about how I have changed his life, or how excited she is to introduce her friends and family to the challenge, and I always take a moment to appreciate how lucky I am to be able to help others learn how to feel their best. But sometimes there are those testimonials that stop me in my tracks; the kind of letters that reinforce every reason for my plan and why I do what I do for a living. I will never forget the day that my dear friend Raymond called me and told me that he was ready to change his life and start his 22-Day Revolution.

Raymond and I had been friends for years, and I had been watching his habits hurt him for all of those years. He has two beautiful children, an amazing wife, and a rewarding career. But his eating habits were catching up with him, and his weight, which had always fluctuated, was going up and up. Raymond was in a downward spiral. When we talked about it, he would admit that he kept mistreating himself over and over, but he somehow couldn't get himself to stop—especially long-term. He would diet and lose some weight, but cash in on the small victories and ultimately end up gaining more weight than he started with. He was at a loss and felt powerless against his own self-proclaimed "irresponsible and destructive habits."

I would encourage him to get more conscious about his eating habits. He would try, but always ended up reverting to his habitual, unhealthy patterns. Raymond is the kind of guy who does everything to the max—he thinks big, works hard, and enjoys life to the fullest. However, what he considered to be "enjoying life" most often meant eating long, decadent meals—usually at restaurants or home parties—and most often accompanied by "fine wine." To him, dieting was a deprivation that meant no longer enjoying himself. What he didn't truly understand was that while he was doing so well in every other aspect of his life, he was using his successes in those areas to justify his poor health habits, and these habits were slowly killing him. From the outside looking in, it made no sense to me that he didn't take control of his health, and it would pain me to watch him neglect himself.

I would say, "Raymond, this is your life we're talking about. Why not capture your success in health as well?"

And Raymond would say, "I know. . . . I'm actually eating better. I was worse before. I'm doing it." But as soon as he would lose a little weight, he would get comfortable, and then gain it back . . . and then some.

Time went by and nothing changed, because there was no habit change and no map for success. Success needs a plan! If you truly want to change, you need to consciously take a good look in the mirror and say, "I can be a better version of myself, and here's how."

When Raymond looked in the mirror, as he expresses, he was in denial. He saw a big guy and was hard on himself, promising to change that day, but when certain clothes masked just how big he felt, he would override his dissatisfaction with his default habits. He began to believe in that image in the mirror; he believed he just needed to accept the way he looked. He told himself that he was just a "big guy." But Raymond was really a slim guy who was around fifty pounds overweight. It was so easy for me, who has experience with physiology, who has seen people transform themselves by changing their eating habits and upping their fitness quotient, to see the real Raymond. The Raymond I imagined was slim and athletic. The Raymond I could see inside the weight was a trim guy who was proud of the way he looked.

But Raymond couldn't see what I saw anymore. He could see his potential, remembering how fit he felt in high school and college. He just didn't believe he could get there again. He could see only that losing that weight would mean cutting out his favorite things—multicourse dinners, bottles of red wine, the works. Raymond kept spiraling, and at five-foot-seven, his weight climbed to over 220 pounds, and his blood pressure hit 151/105 (stage 2 hypertension). Overweight and out of shape, Raymond was seriously putting his health at risk. He was up every night with a rapid heart rate, chest pains, indigestion, and constant heartburn, and his inability to sleep only made him feel worse.

Finally, he hit his rock bottom. Up all night again, unable to sleep again, feeling terrible again, he sat down at the computer one morning and started learning about the potentially fatal effects of high blood pressure and the other symptoms he was experiencing. The more he read, the more he understood how serious his problems were. Angry and frustrated, he agonized about how he could have done this to himself. He couldn't bear the thought of his children losing their dad at a young age, the way he had lost his own father.

That morning, Raymond saw his reflection in the computer screen, looking absolutely defeated and hopeless. Perhaps that was his fate, he thought, and it was all his fault. Then Raymond's son entered the room and saw his father—pale, sick, and stressed.

With worry in his eyes and caution in his voice, his son asked a very simple but poignant question that struck at Raymond's deepest fears and insecurities: "Dad, are you all right?"

Raymond felt as if the air had been sucked out of him. He knew the answer was no. He was not all right. That day he said to his son, "Yes, I'm all right," not wanting him to worry, but for the first time he said no to himself, no to all of the things that were destroying him, and finally started saying yes to the things that would allow him to be a healthy father for as long as he could. He was devastated that his children were watching him destroy his health and that the unhealthy habits they saw from their dad could one day be their own.

It was time to change.

Raymond knew that what he needed was not another crash diet, where he would put a Band-Aid on the problem. He needed to address deep-seated issues and achieve long-term change. That was when he called me.

"If you get on a plant-based program," I told him, "I guarantee that your health problems will go away. You will feel better than ever and become the person you truly are. Do it for you. Do it for your beautiful family."

And then I said the six key words: "Just try it for twenty-two days."

Raymond tried the program, and because of the amount of weight he needed to lose, I suggested he take on the aggressive fast-track program (chapter 15). He stopped drinking alcohol and started eating a plant-based diet, consuming 100 ounces of water a day, and working out daily.

Raymond admits it wasn't like turning on an easy switch and silencing all of his inner demons. As with any lifestyle change, it was harder in the beginning. What kept him from wavering was the thought that he just needed to get past 22 days. Initially he dreaded following through with social plans, knowing that he wouldn't partake in the eating and drinking. After the initial two weeks, his perspective became the exact opposite. Instead of viewing his new way of eating as a deprivation that would balloon until the pressure became so great that he would burst and splurge, it became a liberation that relieved him of his constant battle with himself. He was good with being good.

Ultimately, Raymond made it through 22 days. The result: His blood pressure went down to 120/86 and he lost 22 pounds—how poetic! He continued for another 22 days. After 44 days, his blood pressure went down to 118/77 and he lost over 40 pounds. Today he has lost over 65 pounds! He still eats out at (almost) all the same restaurants several times a week, but orders differently without any hesitation. The most important accomplishment, for Raymond, was realizing that there was no end date. He could keep giving himself the gift of good health day after day, no matter where life took him.

Raymond emerged a changed person from the inside out. He expressed to me his inspiring new outlook, in which sustainable weight loss isn't about racing toward a finish line. It isn't about how long you can endure a demanding struggle. It's about gaining momentum and empowerment with every step forward that you take. Not only is there not an end date, but at 22 days he was just scratching the surface. He started learning things about himself that he had forgotten or never known. He had a greater appreciation for everything he has. He's now in the moment when spending time with loved ones, and has more focus and clarity of thought in his business and creative initiatives.

"Eating plant-based isn't about enjoying yourself less," Raymond told me. "This is about getting the most out of life. It's not about repressing your true desires. It's about unearthing your truest ambitions." Raymond is not an exception, yet rather a prime example that anyone can do it. Many people feel like they can't do it when starting a diet—especially one that, on the surface, feels like a drastic change in the way they eat. However, as with his example, even someone who is a bona fide foodie and has never considered eating vegetarian—let alone vegan—can discover a world of new and inspiring foods. I hoped that Raymond would make it past 22 days and that he would pick up new habits, but I did not imagine he would continue eating vegan (for over a year and counting). The objective of this program is to make changes to your diet that you will incorporate into your life to achieve long-lasting benefits. If you find that after 22 days, there are certain foods that you planned to reintroduce and you don't miss them, don't force them back in. You may be very surprised by what you will accomplish and who you will find within yourself.

THE 22-DAY REVOLUTION PROGRAM

The 22-Day Revolution is a rigorous program designed to overhaul your bad habits and damaged body through a plant-based diet and exercise regimen. By following the program, you'll provide your body with all of the essential vitamins and nutrients you may be missing with a meat-heavy and processed diet, while jump-starting weight loss through portion control and exercise.

5 Guidelines for Your 22-Day Revolution

The 22-Day Revolution meal plan has menus for breakfast, lunch, and dinner. Every single day of your 22-day challenge is fully accounted for, with appealing, simple-to-prepare, plant-based options that you and your family will love. These are the five guidelines you will follow over the next 22 days as you work to reset your body and build new healthy and sustainable habits.

1. Choose Plant-Based over Processed

The more your food looks like it did in nature, the better. Eating whole fruits and vegetables as close to their natural states as possible will enable your body to focus on detoxifying and shedding unhealthy weight, instead of digesting the packaged "Frankenfoods" that compose the average American diet.

Our bodies work overtime to break down and digest them. Processed foods sabotage our overall wellness, damaging our palates and our ability to taste real flavors and often causing stomachaches from all the chemicals and unnatural flavors. With the invention of all of the technology around food production, with the increasing use of artificial flavors and colors, with the mass production of food in huge quantities, our food supply is completely industrialized.

Potato chips are vegan, but they're not good for you. Think about what your great-grandparents ate: whole foods, grown on farms. If your ancestors wouldn't recognize what's on your plate, don't eat it!

2. Eat Three Mindful Meals a Day

Eating to the point of fullness is what makes people gain weight. Listen to your internal cues by eating mindfully—that is, by minimizing outside distractions and sitting calmly at a table, focusing on how your body feels. The goal of this program is to be sustainable and to really work for you and your life. I want you to succeed! That's why I've designed the program so that you eat three meals a day: breakfast, lunch, and dinner. Because that's how your family eats, and how your colleagues eat—and because it works!

Eat dinner at least two hours before you go to sleep. We eat calories to give us energy to move through our day. Your body will benefit from time to digest before you sleep. And no midnight snacks!

The key to eating well and not gaining weight is to eat with restraint. The absolute healthiest way to eat is to 80 percent fullness, or just a little bit less than full. While on the program, follow the portions outlined. If you've been overeating for years, or are more than fifty pounds overweight, the portions outlined in the 22-day program will feel small. This may feel uncomfortable at first if you've become accustomed to that "too full" feeling, but as your body (and mind) adjusts, you'll feel more energized after meals. That's why the plan allows for healthy snacks as needed. But also remember that this is a 22-day intensive program to reset your body and mind. It will be challenging, but as your body adjusts to the correct portion sizes, you'll learn what 80 percent fullness should feel like.

And you'll realize that eating until you're stuffed is an uncomfortable way of eating, because it makes you feel bloated and heavy instead of light and energized.

3. Aim for 80-10-10 (80 Percent Carbohydrates, 10 Percent Fat, 10 Percent Protein)

It may seem crazy in this world of trendy low-carb diets, but when the carbs you're eating are fresh and whole and come directly from the earth, then you can eat them in abundance. A plant-based diet includes nutritious, complex carbs found in fresh fruits and vegetables, as well as within most protein sources, like legumes. When you're eating plants, you don't have to obsess about calories. For a healthy diet, I suggest a breakdown of 80 percent carbohydrates, 10 percent fat, 10 percent protein. And that's easy on a plant-based diet, because fruits and vegetables are naturally full of complex carbohydrates and low in fat.

If you're looking to fast-track your weight loss, keep in mind that although all vegetables and grains are good sources of complex carbs, some are a better choice for daytime meals than evening meals. Quinoa has a greater balance of complex carbs than carrots, and legumes contain more carbs than broccoli or cauliflower. So when you're eating for weight loss, during the 22-Day Revolution program, I suggest eating heavier carbs like quinoa during the day instead of at night. If you really want to lose the weight quickly, include grains and legumes with breakfast and lunch, ensuring that your body has ample opportunity to utilize this energy during the day. By skipping heavier carbs at dinnertime, you'll give your body a chance to work off of fat stores for needed energy overnight.

You don't need to eat animals in order to get all of your vitamins and minerals—including and especially protein! The idea that you might not get enough protein on a vegan or vegetarian diet is a common misconception. Think about it: Where did all the nutrition in the animals you have been eating come from? Plants! Plants are the original source of all the minerals in the animals you have been consuming.

4. Exercise for 30 Minutes Each Day

Exercise counts. It's essential to creating the healthy balance that we all need in order to feel our best. It's an essential component of the 22-Day Revolution program, and especially important if you're looking to lose weight. Yes, diet counts, and it counts big. But the supporting cast matters too. If you want real results, once you've got your diet balanced, you'll want to do whatever you can to help yourself. Eating plants will reset your body: exercise will make sure the reset sticks.

Remember that doing one doesn't excuse you from the other. Diet doesn't excuse you from exercise, and exercise doesn't give you carte blanche to indulge. Successful weight loss is 75 percent diet and 25 percent exercise. You can never outwork the damage done by a bad diet, so exercise for health rather than as an excuse to eat. Once you exercise and feel the positive effects of natural endorphins, you're more likely to embrace healthy foods and have the strength to resist temptation.

To complement your eating and increase the benefits of a plant-based diet—energy, weight loss, and vitality—make sure to work out every day for at least thirty minutes.

5. Drink Water, aka Don't Drink Your Calories

Water is best. Unsweetened teas are great; so is water with lemon. Leave soda behind, skip the sugary teas and lemonade, and remember that sugary drinks and alcohol contain empty calories that will sabotage your best efforts on this program.

The eight-glasses-per-day rule may be a bit simplistic. The Institute of Medicine suggests that men drink 13 eight-ounce cups and women drink nine eight-ounce cups a day.[4] Start the day with a glass of water and lemon. This is good for alkalinity, digestion, and rehydration.

Here are a few tips to help you manage fluid intake throughout the day:

- Drink a glass of water/fluid with each meal
- Drink a glass of water/fluid between each meal
- Drink a glass of water/fluid before, during, and after exercise
- Drink more water/fluid when it's hot
- Don't wait until you're thirsty to drink water; once you are thirsty you are likely dehydrated

If you're exercising and sweating, you'll need to take in more fluid to compensate. The more your body weighs, the greater your need for water. The best way to find out if you are getting enough water daily is to observe your body. First, you should be urinating regularly, and your urine should be colorless or a light yellow. Dark yellow urine is a sign of dehydration. It may not be the most fun to take a look, but it's the best indicator. Other signs of overall dehydration are dark circles or bags under your eyes, flaky skin or acne, a dry and red nose, headaches, and a dry mouth.

When your body is properly hydrated you should have more energy, and your skin and hair will appear more lustrous. Being properly

---

[4] http://www.mayoclinic.org/healthy-living/nutrition-and-healthy-eating/in-depth/water/art-20044256?pg=1, accessed September 3, 2014.

hydrated can help reduce wrinkles (by plumping up your skin cells), give you stronger hair and nails, even reduce hangover and sunburn effects. Drinking a glass or two of water before a meal can curb overeating and help you feel full between meals.

What you'll learn over the course of the program:

By following the simple rules listed above, you're going to change your entire relationship with the food you eat, for the better. You're going to learn how to think about the big picture, about how you want to feel in the long run, not just this moment. You'll learn to identify the true feeling of fullness, so that you can stop eating when your body has had enough. You'll see that you can eat healthfully without counting calories, just by eating plants, eating consciously, and stopping when you're full. And you'll see that you can lose the weight and keep it off by transitioning from a yo-yo lifestyle to a sustainable, simple, yet enriching way of eating.

When I say simple, I mean it! Eating well and losing weight doesn't need to be hard. Once you're accustomed to eating food from the earth, dieting is something you'll no longer need to think about. The hard work on this program is changing your habits from unconsciously eating processed food throughout the day to mindfully eating plant-based meals. Once plants are your habit, the journey is easy! That's because nature knows best. Plant-based food is perfectly designed to sustain us. When you follow the daily menus on this program, you don't have to count calories or macronutrients, because the right balance is built into the menus. That will train your body to become accustomed to how it really feels to eat the right foods. After the program, you'll be ready to take it to the next level—and you still won't have to count calories or macronutrients. Once you know your habits are transformed, eating a variety of plants will naturally give you the healthy balance of 80-10-10, and listening to your internal cues will keep you from eating too much at mealtimes. Sustainable weight loss will be inevitable!

WHAT DOES PLANT-BASED REALLY MEAN?

The 22-Day Revolution plan is totally suitable for vegans, because it is vegan! We call this plant-based eating instead of vegan because that's what it's about: eating plants. A truly plant-based diet is vegan, but a vegan diet is not necessarily plant-based. You can be a vegan and live on potato chips, pretzels, and vegan hot dogs served on gluten-free bread. But these processed foods can make you just as sick and unhealthy as a meat-inclusive diet, and they are not part of a plant-based diet!

Vegetarian: Eats milk and eggs, grains, vegetables. Doesn't eat meat, poultry, fish.

Vegan: Doesn't eat meat, poultry, fish, milk, eggs, honey. Eats grains, vegetables, fruit, or overprocessed vegan foods.

Plant-based: Eats 100 percent plants: grains, vegetables, fruit. Doesn't eat meat, poultry, fish, milk, eggs, or processed vegan foods.

Remember, just because something doesn't contain meat does not mean that it is plant-based! If you are eating a vegan hot dog made in a vegan bun made from processed flours, you may be a vegan, but you are *not* on the 22-Day Revolution program. When we say plant-based, we mean plants, not food made in a plant. We mean a diet that consists of 100 percent delicious foods that come from the earth.

We mean a diet of food that will make us feel our best, today and every day that follows.

WHY I EAT PLANTS

I consider myself to be lucky, because my own awareness of the connection between the food we eat and the way we feel began when I was very young. Of course, as a child, I ate what my parents ate. In my Cuban family, food was a central part of our family gatherings, a way for my mother to show her love for us all. The food I learned to eat was the food that was available in my home and my community. That's how it works: our earliest habits are learned unconsciously. But as we grow and have our own experiences and become more aware, we may realize that the habits we have learned do not really work for us.

That's the realization I had one morning, on the way to school, when I ate a pastry, not something I had ever thought very much about. Eating a pastry was not taboo in my community or in my family—it was just a pastry. But then something funny happened—my body rebelled against what I was feeding it in the mornings and I got an angry rash on my arm. I tried to ignore it but it kept getting worse. My arm was itchy and swollen, I couldn't concentrate on my work, and I had to go to the nurse, and then my mom had to come pick me up early, which meant that she had to miss work. And that was a very big deal; she was a single parent and I was very conscious that her job was very important for my family.

The last thing I wanted to do was cause my mom any stress, so I thought very hard about what might have caused the rash. Then the nurse had asked whether I had any allergies, and I knew the only thing I had eaten that day was the pastry, and that led me to make the first important connection—that eating bad food causes problems. So I decided to do what I could to avoid the problem and not cause my mom any more stress: I stopped eating pastries. Unfortunately for me, I hadn't yet made the second connection—that we must eat good food if we want to thrive! So instead of eating pastries, I ate nothing for breakfast. I went to school hungry, which of course led to my feeling listless and not having enough energy—until a week later, when I passed out in PE class. That was when I made the second connection! Pastries didn't work, but skipping breakfast was equally ineffective.

My journey began at that moment. I started to listen to my body and began learning everything I could about nutrition and fitness, and all of these years later, what I know is that balanced nutrition is the basis of feeling good about ourselves physically, emotionally, and mentally. I've been eating plant-based for nearly a decade, but the change didn't happen overnight. First I gave up dairy. That felt so good I stopped eating chicken, and then eggs. The more I learned, the more I leaned toward plant-based—and I've never felt better! The last thing to go was fish.

After nearly two decades of working with clients as an exercise physiologist, I was in top physical shape and I maintained a pescetarian diet—meaning I ate only fish. I allowed myself fish because I thought it would be very difficult to eat plant-based all the time while out to eat and traveling, without resorting to processed foods. Then I noticed it was more of an excuse than it needed to be. Instead of seeking out the healthiest option and putting in the extra effort that would result in my eating the kind of food I wanted to be eating, I would order fish. The truth is that most of the fish we eat out (this was the only time I was eating fish) is farmed. Research has shown farmed fish to have less usable heart-healthy omega-3 and a lower protein content; they're fattier, with higher levels of omega-6 (an imbalance of omega-3 and omega-6 can cause inflammation in the body); and cancer-causing PCBs exist in farmed salmon at much higher rates than in wild salmon. I knew I could do better.

I've always been in search of optimal wellness. I love to educate myself about nutrition, and the more I learned about plant-based nutrition, the more I knew that it was the very best way to feed and fuel your body. I like to challenge myself, so I finally took the opportunity to change my diet.

Going plant-based led to a ton of questions from everyone around me. Why would I go plant-based when I didn't need to lose weight? It was true that I felt good before I made the switch, and while I never had health issues like high blood pressure or high cholesterol, there is a history of heart disease in my family, so I thought I was ensuring myself against future problems. Even with my strong health profile, making the shift to plant-based led to some eye-opening results.

During my first year eating plant-based, even though I maintained the same weight, there were some meaningful benefits. I travel a lot for business, and I would occasionally get sick from travel. That stopped happening. Another main difference was that I immediately noticed my recovery time from my workouts getting shorter and shorter, to the point where now, my recovery time was almost nonexistent. This improvement has been incredibly important to my athletic development, and I love that I can push myself further. Any aches and pains, joint wear from tough workouts and overuse, decreased in frequency until they basically stopped altogether. A year after beginning to eat plant-based, I went for my physical and routine blood tests. My inflammation markers were so low they were barely detectable (inflammation is the underlying cause of many age-related diseases). My already low cholesterol levels were even better than before.

My doctor asked what I was doing differently, and I was happy to tell him that my shift to a plant-based diet had been more effective than I had ever dreamed possible.

In the beginning, this diet was sometimes difficult to maintain when I traveled. But it wasn't impossible. When you really want something, you can make it happen no matter what. For example, when I'm traveling to a conference and I know the food they're serving isn't what's best for my body, I do my research. I'll try to find a hotel located near a shopping center or town that has a Whole Foods or other supermarket with a wide selection. When I arrive in town, I'll stop in to pick up some water and healthy plant-based snacks for my room, and I'll return as needed to get food for my meals. I know I can find what I need at Whole Foods, and I know I'll feel better if I prioritize my health, so I put myself in a position to succeed.

Now, after nearly a decade of eating a plant-based diet, I feel better than ever—energetic and strong.

And so can you.

2

POSITIVE HABITS CREATE
A POSITIVE LIFE

HOW DID YOU FEEL WHEN you got up this morning? Did you wake up feeling incredible? Were you full of energy, joy, and gratitude for your healthy and strong body? Did you sit up in bed, stretch, and think to yourself, *This is going to be another amazing day!*

If not, if you woke up feeling sluggish and exhausted, wishing you could sleep just a little bit more, knowing that even if you did, you'd still be tired when you crawled out of bed . . . then something isn't right.

Your habits—what you eat and drink, whether or not you exercise, how much sleep you get—are responsible for how you feel when you get into bed at night and how you feel when you wake up in the morning. So if you're accustomed to feeling lousy instead of incredible, if you think it's "normal" to feel under the weather instead of over the moon, if you think it's "normal" to drag yourself around all day instead of bouncing from place to place—I'd like to introduce you to a new normal. A normal where you wake up feeling revived. Where you finish a meal and feel powered up instead of weighed down. Where getting on the scale is something you look forward to, because it confirms what you already knew: that your habits are leading you towards achieving your goals, just like they should.

Why keep making choices that just lead to feeling bad? Why eat food that makes you feel fat and sick? Nobody wants to feel bad! Do you want to feel healthy, vital, and powerful? Of course you do. We all do. *Anyone* can do it. And *everyone* should.

WHY SOME PEOPLE ARE MORE SUCCESSFUL THAN OTHERS

When I was young, I was always curious about the behaviors that lead to success—success in sports, success in health, success in the way we look and feel. Why was it that some people were able to have great muscle tone and consistent energy and verve, while others seemed tired and sad and were visibly overweight? Why would some of my fellow athletes go on to win championships while others fumbled and quit? Why can some people completely turn their lives around while others struggle with the same problems again and again?

I began to notice one common behavior consistent with success, and that was the presence of positive habits. Making positive choices led to positive results. Interestingly, successful people were often aware of what their habits were, while unsuccessful people seemed unaware that their habits were controlling them.

The winners seemed to possess the awareness that actions have consequences, and that by choosing specific actions, they could reap the rewards they wanted. They were able to consciously choose a goal, determine what steps would get them to their goal, and then follow through. Unsuccessful people seemed to think that success just happens, or that some people were born with an ability to succeed and that others were not.

I realized that being successful wasn't about who you were or where you were born—it was about being conscious and aware that the choices you make on a daily basis really affect you in the long run. They either get you to the championships, or they keep you on the sidelines.

As I got older my curiosity and interest only grew, and as a result I pursued a degree in exercise physiology, and I chose what I call a proactive approach to health and wellness by becoming a personal trainer and subsequently a lifestyle coach—and what I learned along the way only made the view clearer! Our habits are the basis for our success—or our failure. If you want to be the best at anything (including the best version of yourself), you have to have systems in place for success. These systems are healthy habits!

The truth is that no matter who you are or how much money you have or how little, whether you have five children or none, whether you are a man or a woman, whether you are young or old, you have habits—those little things you do every day, all the time, whether you're thinking about it or not. They are the actions that got you where you are.

MAKE BETTER HABITS INSTEAD OF EXCUSES

Everybody has an excuse for why they aren't reaching their goals. "My entire family is overweight." "I just love junk food." "I'm a couch potato!" "I have a sweet tooth." "I just love food." "I'd rather watch a football game than play one." "I hate vegetables."

All of those stories are, at root, the same. They are all about personal habits. The habits of heavy parents become the habits of heavy children. Junk food is a habit. TV is a habit. Laziness is a habit. And these habits have dire consequences, but they all have solutions and can all be reversed.

For most of my life, I've been hearing that a great deal of disease is hereditary—but the data shows otherwise. For example, when it comes to risk for heart disease, cancer, stroke, and diabetes, the leading causes of disease have been linked to many lifestyle factors. What exactly are lifestyle factors, and how do we learn them? We learn them from watching those closest to us, often our families.

Eating processed foods or eating plants begins as a choice, but ultimately, it becomes a habit. Over the past decade, I have cultivated the habits of eating the gorgeous, bountiful, vibrant foods that the earth gives us. I eat the plants that make our planet beautiful and also give us the best nutrition we can possibly get. I eat fruits and vegetables that maximize my energy and my health. I eat food that cuts my risk of diabetes, heart disease, and obesity, diseases that so many people today are getting because they eat too much processed food. For many of those people, those processed foods are no longer a choice. They are a habit—a habit that is ruining lives, ruining health and sabotaging success.

If you are overweight, unhealthy habits are the culprit. If you want to change your lifestyle, if you want to change your life, you have to start with your habits.

THE FORCE OF HABITS

When I was in college, I studied psychology and habit formation. Our habits are the mechanisms that make us tick, like a program in a computer. In an effort to make you more efficient, your brain helps out by building pathways based on the things you do again and again, making it easier to repeat that action. Habits let you run on automatic, making energy-saving choices for you while you barely notice. When you brush your teeth, are you focusing on moving your arm up and down? More likely you've already brushed your teeth so many times that you don't need to be mentally present, so you're brushing and rinsing and putting the toothbrush away while you're thinking about what you need to accomplish for the day, or what you're going to wear. Have you ever driven a route you drive all the time, and when you arrive you aren't quite sure how you got there? Your habits took over so that your mind could think about other things. But you were still actively making decisions along the way, even though you didn't realize it!

Even when you set your car to cruise control, if you're approaching danger, you can still step on the brake and slow things down. You can still turn the wheel.

Let's look at your morning routine. How often do you turn off the alarm, get out of bed, shower, get dressed, and head out the door on autopilot? What we do most often is what we are most comfortable doing, and eventually it requires little to no active decision making. A habitual action is based on past learning; it's the result of choices you made over the past days and weeks and months, not the result of a choice made consciously today.

Your entire life, the sum of who you are, can be reduced to your habits. In another way of looking at it, if you add up all your habits, you get to exactly where you are right now. If you are the sum of your habits, then isn't it time to make a conscious decision about making them the healthiest and most beneficial choices possible? It's time to wake up from the unconscious, passive role you're taking in your life and make informed changes.

The more often you make a choice, the more likely it is that you will continue to make that choice, and the more likely you will become less and less aware that you ever made that choice to begin with.

Hundreds of times day, probably thousands of times, you make choices that impact your health. From brushing and flossing to getting physical activity to every bite of food you do or do not put into your mouth, your choices have an effect on your overall well-being. The odds are that, over time, you aren't conscious of most of those choices, because they have become automated. They have become habits.

This insight is at the core of your 22-Day Revolution.

If you are to succeed—and the goal of this program is success—then you are going to have to identify your habits and consciously change them. And you're going to work to slowly, carefully make sure those changes stick.

CAN HABITS REALLY BE CHANGED?

Habits can absolutely be changed. The area of your brain located around your forehead is called your prefrontal cortex, and it is where most of the thinking and planning you do happens. Although habits have long been thought of as automatic, and for the most part they are, a recent MIT study demonstrated that there is a small part of your prefrontal cortex that retains moment-by-moment control of the actions being exercised.[5] Even when you don't know it, even if you've never exercised it, even if you've never heard of your prefrontal cortex, it is still hard at work for you.

We all know people who do the things they say they will do. If you see them at a party and they say they are buying a new house, within weeks you hear that they are having a housewarming party. If they tell you that they are going to lose thirty pounds, when you see them a few months later, they are about to hike up Mount Kilimanjaro to celebrate their new muscular physique. If they mention that they mean to learn to knit, within weeks you get a handmade scarf-and-hat set in the mail.

How does that happen? It happens because those people have made the connection between the little actions we take every day and what we wind up accomplishing over the long run. They already know—without knowing that they know—that there's a part of their prefrontal cortex keeping them in the driver's seat.

[5] http://newsoffice.mit.edu/2012/understanding-how-brains-control-our-habits-1029, accessed June 25, 2014.

Do you want to be the kind of person who accomplishes the things you want to do? Of course, we all want to create the life we want to live, and accomplish our goals and dreams. A key factor of success is awareness. Successful people know what their habits are and how those habits are affecting their lives, while unsuccessful people seem unaware that their habits are controlling them. Instead of talking about what you're going to do—do it! Take one small step at a time, and day by day you'll build the positive habits that will help you reach your goals. Making positive choices leads to positive results!

HABITS FOR HEALTH

If you want to lose weight or if you're suffering from a major health issue, like cardiovascular disease or diabetes, let's take a closer look at the habits that got you there.

Your habits are everything. A steady drip of water will eventually carve stone. That extra dessert, your candy-corn addiction, the bowl of M&M's on your desk: All of these are cumulative health bombs, practically invisible one by one, but powerful enough to ruin your health if you let them. Whether or not you always order chocolate cake, if you reward yourself every afternoon with a handful of candies, these are the habits that got you where you are.

When you really look closely, our lives are a cluster of habits that we practice on a daily basis in almost the same way every time. Change the habits, change the outcome.

If you're worried about weight and you eat a doughnut for breakfast every morning, shift that habit and eat a bowl of chia and oatmeal. That simple switch would give you a burst of energy that lasts all morning, and a host of vitamins and minerals (including the omegas everyone's always talking about) to help your body run more efficiently. Small change, big results.

What are your habits doing for you—or to you? What are they pushing you toward—or keeping you from?

In just 22 days, you can change those negative habits, and usher in not just the rest of your life, but the best of your life. You can be healthier, more energetic, and more productive. You can feel great instead of "okay." You can feel powerful instead of "fine." And you can start living the life you want, not just the one you have, right now, today, with the help of the 22-Day Revolution.

You will learn how to eat more fruits and vegetables and whole grains. You will learn how to eat mindfully and the optimal amount to feel your best. You will experience the benefits of eating foods rich in vitamins and minerals, giving you energy and vitality you haven't felt in years. You will redefine your relationship with food, because as you practice restraint, you will enjoy your food like never before. You will find the strength to change your life, and through the hard work you put in, you will find a renewed sense of confidence in what you can accomplish when the goal is really worth it.

I'm not saying that it's going to be easy. Starting a revolution means having to do some fighting! You're fighting against a lifetime of ingrained habits of overeating, overindulging. How many times have you pushed back from the table with a stomachache because you kept reaching for seconds and thirds and fourths? You thought that you were indulging, but you were really building unhealthy habits that would hurt you in the long run.

As you recondition your body to eat the right foods in the right amounts, you're going to have to work hard to get used to the way full really feels. And to you, it is possible that it will feel like being hungry, because you have learned to associate nausea with fullness. But nauseous doesn't feel like full. It feels like overindulgence.

Do you know what real indulgence gives you? *Power!* When you feed yourself a gorgeous plant-based meal, and you eat the right amount, as soon as you get over the fact that you don't feel sick or like you need to lie down or unbuckle your belt, you realize that you aren't actually hungry. What you are is satisfied.

But please don't be frustrated if it takes a little while for your stomach and your mind to catch up to where you're going. If you're used to a sensation of overfullness, once you have eaten the right amount of food for you, you may think you want a little more. But please hang on. Try. Give it twenty minutes. Take a walk. Have a glass of water or a cup of tea. Keep it up and keep it going. Because when you get a sense of the way real indulgence feels, when you realize that you can enjoy delicious food without guilt or shame, that you can eat well and still lose weight— well, that's the biggest reward of all.

The food you eat can either be the thing that keeps you from achieving your goals—or it can be what gets you to your goals. You have the power! No matter what your habits have been, no matter how you define yourself, I'm here to tell you that it is possible. It is doable. You can stop letting other people define you! You can stop letting your past choices define you!

It's time to allow newer, stronger, healthier habits and actions to define you.

3

PLANTS RULE

ONE MORNING, MY SON SAW me drinking a green juice, and he said, "Papi, what is that? I want some."

I said, "I don't think you'll like it."

He said, "Why?"

"Because it doesn't taste really good. It's really, really strong. And it's only for grown-ups, because it gives you big muscles."

He said, "I want big muscles."

"Yeah, but you're not going to be able to drink it, because it doesn't taste good."

"I can drink it."

"I don't know; it's for grown-ups."

"I want it."

I said, "Okay. Here."

He drank it and said, "Aaaaargh!" and made a terrible face. Then he said, "Let me have some more. . . . Aargh. Let me have some more." He drank the whole glass—it was his first green drink, and it had everything in it except the kitchen sink. It was so bitter, but he was fine with it, because he saw it as a tool to get those big muscles his heroes have. And now he drinks green juice all the time.

So I learned to do the same thing with all the kids I encounter who are curious about healthy eating! I've gone to my kids' school and I've made great green drinks that are totally yummy, with lots of fruit, and I'll let them have the ones that taste like fruit punch.

And then I say, "Okay, who's ready for something brave?"

And they all say, "Me, me, me."

Appreciation of health isn't about how old we are. It's about how receptive we are to learning new things. Everybody can learn to eat plants and love it! Whatever habits you learned from your parents or your friends when you were young, no matter what you think you love to eat, you can learn to love eating plants.

As soon as you take those first steps, you'll see the enormous benefits right away. For me, that's the real basis of this book, and of everything I do. I am so grateful that the messages I put into the world about eating vegan and loving plant-based foods are embraced by my children as well as my clients and my friends, because eating plants has an impact on every part of your life. There's a certain kind of empowerment that comes from eating better, from feeling better, from looking better. It affects you on such a deep level—emotionally, spiritually—that you have energy to be kinder to the people around you. When you put good food into your body, you feel better about yourself. The better you feel, the easier it is to offer kindness to other people and accept the kindness of others. Good feelings are contagious! When you feel good, others feel good. When you share your inner joy with the world, every person you come into contact with feels a little bit more joyous.

Consciousness about what we eat starts with wanting to make ourselves whole and healthy—and winds up turning you into the kind of person who wants to make others feel whole and healthy, too.

EATING PLANTS IS GOOD FOR THE WHOLE FAMILY

I've always taught my children that if you want to live a happy and healthy life, if you want to have energy, you must eat nutritious and satisfying foods and get plenty of exercise. And you know what? Kids love it. They love eating well and knowing that they are helping themselves grow up to be healthy and strong.

Recently, my son's class did a project in school to help them answer the familiar question "What do you want to be when you grow up?" Some of the kids said "doctor" and some said "police officer" or "teacher" or "astronaut." My son's poster board said, "Nutritionist."

I could not have been a prouder dad at that moment. Seeing my son embrace these ideas for himself makes me as happy as I could possibly be, because I know that good nutrition leads to a long, healthy,[6] and fulfilling life. Studies show that children who are raised as vegetarians have a lower BMI than their meat-eating compatriots. As they grow into adolescence, the difference only becomes greater. The message is that eating plants is healthy for children and for adults.

As infants, children naturally stop eating when they are full. But as they get older, they learn from whatever they are exposed to. Teach them healthy habits and they will crave healthy food. Give them too much sugar, and that's what they'll crave. Remember the old saying, "Kids learn from what we show them, not what we tell them"? The choices that lead to disease or risk of disease are learned behaviors! These learned behaviors, whether we are talking about diet or inactivity, are all habits we develop as kids that stay with us as adults.

In my experience, kids who have been exposed to healthy foods and taught how important they are for our bodies love to eat plants, because they love to feel like they are taking good care of themselves. But they have to learn it somewhere! Too many adults make excuses for children's desires for sugary, processed foods, just like they make excuses for themselves. They indulge their own desire to overeat and do not eat with restraint, which leads to a relationship with food mired in guilt instead of joy. It starts with the adults! Parents are the first teachers for their children, providing the tools and skills they need to make healthy choices and live a life of health and vitality—or not. Whenever I see overweight parents eating huge portions of unhealthy foods, I see children who are overweight and have the same habits as the parents. When I see families where the parents hike and play sports and are conscious about health, the children have the same habits.

Habits are just as hereditary as genetic risk of disease. If you got the wrong messages as a child and you never developed those good habits, you already know what the repercussions of poor eating are: weight gain, bad skin, bad health, bad moods. If you want to have optimal health at any age, choose a plant-based diet!

---

[6] J. Sabaté and M.J, Wien, M. "Vegetarian Diets and Childhood Obesity Prevention." *Am J Clin Nutr.* May 2010; 91 (5):1525S–1529S. DOI: http://dx.doi.org/10.3945/ajcn.2010.28701F. [PubMed].

Teaching our children the best way to eat and to fuel their bodies for success is paramount. About one in three American kids and teens is overweight or obese. Childhood obesity is now the number one health concern among parents in the United States, topping drug abuse and smoking. And soon we may see the first generation that will have a shorter life expectancy than their parents.[7] Let's stop this trend and reverse the effects of the overindulgent, overprocessed diet we're feeding our kids and eating ourselves. As you saw from my own son, kids want to follow their parents. So in helping yourself create new, healthy habits for a plant-based diet, you're not only changing your life, you're changing the lives of your children.

EATING PLANTS IS GOOD FOR US AND FOR THE PLANET

I chose a plant-based diet for completely selfish reasons: because I've always been in search of optimal wellness, and everything I learned and read pointed me in this direction. The fact is that eating plant-based is just better for you as an individual. Once I started experiencing all the benefits, I was able to see that the side effects of these great choices had their benefits: eating plants isn't just better for me, it's better for the whole world.

It was only as a result of my desire for personal wellness that I stumbled into a cruelty-free lifestyle that made me realize the echoes of my choices were much more profound than I ever imagined. The fact is that we are living in an age in which, despite all of our technology and advancements, our environment is at risk, and people around the world are still starving.

Plants are a superior food source for humans, for their nutrition and also for their impact. For us as individuals and collectively, as a group, eating plants just makes more sense than eating animals. Consider that plants yield ten times more protein per acre than meat. And that one acre of land can produce 20,000 pounds of potatoes or 165 pounds of beef.[8]

---

[7] http://www.heart.org/HEARTORG/GettingHealthy/Overweight-in-Children_UCM_304054_Article.jsp, accessed September 15, 2014.

[8] John Robbins, *Diet for a New America.*

Since plants are nutrient-dense, we could grow more food in less space for more people. That means a lot when you consider that approximately 870 million people in the world do not eat enough to be healthy.[9]

And a plant-based diet is better for the planet. The amount of beef the average American eats in a year creates as much greenhouse gas as driving a car more than 1,800 miles. In addition, the United Nations' Food and Agriculture Organization estimates that the meat industry generates nearly one-fifth of the man-made greenhouse-gas emissions that are accelerating climate change worldwide . . . far more than transportation.[10]

But awareness is rising! According to the 2014 "Vegetarians in America" study conducted by the *Vegetarian Times*, seven million Americans are already vegetarians, one million of those are completely vegan, and more than 23 million people are "vegetarian-inclined."

In a world that is quickly becoming smaller, it's vital that we take a look at how our food consumption is affecting the environment. If eating plants can make us feel better every single day while it reduces or minimizes world hunger and global warming, why wouldn't we embrace it?

For myself, I take great pride in knowing that the long-term effects of my decision to go plant-based will not only protect my health and the health of this planet but also provide an example for my children to follow.

FOOD COUNTS MORE THAN EXERCISE

As an exercise physiologist, I appreciate more than most the importance of exercise in creating a healthy lifestyle. And yet, diet more than exercise accounts for your health and, importantly, your weight, a fact I have proven time and again with my clients. Successful weight loss is 75 percent diet and 25 percent exercise. You can't work off the damage that processed meats do so please, exercise for health instead of as an excuse to eat. If you want to lose the weight and change your health, you must develop the healthy habit of eating plants.

[9] World Food Programme via 22daysnutrition.com.

[10] Meatless Monday via 22daysnutrition.com.

Eating plants can help reverse the symptoms of some major diseases. It can also prevent disease in the first place! I began my career with the goal of helping to prevent disease by changing habits, a proactive approach to health that's easier than treating disease symptoms with prescriptions and drugs. I knew the keys to my own athletic success and healthy physique were rooted in the food I ate, and I wanted to share the message of empowerment that my clients could control their health and well-being by simply changing their diet. I loved working with people as they implemented these small changes in their daily lives, and watching as their confidence and joy in life grew as they became the best possible version of themselves.

I had been training clients on a one-to-one basis for a number of years in Miami, and I wanted to take my business to the next level. The best form of cardio is short, intense workouts, and I found a particularly effective high-intensity workout in spinning. So I decided to open the first spinning studio in Miami.

Spinning was not as well-known in the early nineties as it is now. I remember people saying, "Bicycles in a room? That doesn't make any sense. Who wants to ride a bike in a room?" Nonetheless, I felt it would be awesome, a high-intensity workout in just 45 minutes, and with the camaraderie of a group, but a workout based on individual performance. I went all in and invested in opening the studio. The day I opened the doors, I took a good look at my checkbook—I had spent everything on this opportunity. There was no turning back. I had to make it work.

At the beginning it was just me. I was the instructor. I was the receptionist. I was teaching eight classes a day. I would open the door, let people in, charge them, get on the bike, teach the class, get off the bike, open the door, let them out, let a group of people in, charge them, over and over and over again.

Word got around. Within a month every class was full. There was a waiting list. It was just amazing.

The bikes had come to south Florida. People loved it!

As I developed a really loyal fan base, some members were especially enthusiastic. A particular group of women all came to class together; they were beautiful women who were a little overweight, perhaps 30 pounds. And then they started coming twice a day.

And I thought to myself, *Oh, my God, this is going to be huge.* These were incredible women, and it was so gratifying to see them in my classes every day. I was working hard, and so were they, and I knew our partnership was going to benefit all of us. They were going to lose the weight they wanted to lose, and I was going to get the satisfaction of helping people achieve their transformations, just as I had set out to do. I was so excited! They would feel and look incredible, and they would tell their friends this was how they lost the weight. . . . I couldn't wait to see these women transform their lives. They were so committed to the classes that I just knew it would be the first time in their lives that they had so much success with an exercise program.

A week went by, and then two weeks, and then a month, but the transformations I was waiting for didn't come.

The women were still working out with me twice a day, but they looked exactly the same. And I thought, *This doesn't make any sense. What is going on here?*

Once I turned on my analytical brain and started looking for a solution, I realized that it all came down to habits. My clients had developed a habit for exercise, but they had never created a habit around eating healthy. They were completely unconscious about what they were putting into their bodies, and it was derailing them.

And their habit of working out wasn't about exercising and getting results. It was about socializing. They all got together at nine a.m. to take my class and laugh and talk with one another, and then after carpool, they would come back and exercise again, but they weren't thinking about exercising. They were spending time together and having fun.

They were definitely breaking a sweat in my classes—that was for sure, and they knew it. Since their habit was about fun and not about results, and since all that exercise made them feel like they were burning so many calories in my classes that they could eat whatever they wanted in their brunches, they hadn't been able to lose a pound. They were eating more than they were burning, and the weight was never going to come off unless the way they ate changed. I knew I could help them achieve their goals, but of course I didn't want to offend them.

Ultimately, if they were coming to classes, I had a responsibility to help them achieve the full benefits. I wanted them to have the transformation that was easily within their reach.

So I came up with a plan. I approached them after class one day and asked them whether they would help me with a study I was creating. They all agreed, with their usual great enthusiasm, and I explained what the program I would put them on would do.

"I'm challenging the way we look at exercise and diet. I want to see how much more effective exercise is when you eat plant-based nutrition."

Just like I'm challenging you, I challenged the ladies to shift their food focus to healthy, clean, organic, plant-based foods—fruit, vegetables, grains. I asked them to leave off all the processed foods they were used to eating, and the fast foods, and the steaks, and the cheesesteaks, and the . . . You get the picture. Instead of a table full of the foods that were causing all their health and weight problems, I challenged them to set their tables with green vegetables, root vegetables, quinoa, brown rice, beans, apples, pears, watermelon, and other amazing fresh foods. As Michael Pollan says, "If it came from a plant, eat it; if it was made in a plant, don't."

I knew that if they followed the plan, they would see results. I told them that once they adjusted to this new style of eating, they would no longer crave dead, overprocessed foods, but they would also experience increased energy levels, improved sleep, better moods, and reduced body fat. They would lose weight, and they would get healthier.

This was an amazing experience for me, because I was really putting together all the things I had worked so hard to study: psychology, physiology, anatomy, and nutrition.

Over the next few weeks, the women followed my menus, eating vegetables and fruit and grains. They cooked more at home. They prepared and shared their salads with one another instead of indulging in gourmet brunches full of saturated fat, processed carbs, and all the other things their bodies did not want. They did not eat their regular meals of processed, stripped flours, meat, chicken, fish, cheese, or eggs. They ate fresh fruits, vibrant veggies, gorgeous grains, and do you know what happened?

Results happened.

In just a few weeks, these women—who had been exercising twice a day for a month with no weight loss—began to shed the pounds they longed to and became the healthiest, happiest versions of themselves. By changing their eating habits, they achieved success. Combined, they lost one hundred pounds in six weeks.

They all transformed.
Every single one of them.
By eating plants.

REAL FOODS HAVE REAL FLAVORS AND REAL BENEFITS

"I never thought I could have this much energy."

"My stomach doesn't hurt anymore."

"I never thought it would be so delicious."

"All my friends want to try it now."

These are some of the typical comments I get from people who have transitioned to a plant-based diet. So many of us have become accustomed to feeling tired and nauseated, bloated and listless on a daily basis.

When you become accustomed to eating all of these Frankenfoods instead of real foods, you become so used to the artificial burst of fake flavor that when you taste a real flavor, your taste buds don't know what to do. It's like you've had so much artificial lemon flavor that your taste buds are confused by the natural citric bite of a real lemon, so much artificial cherry flavoring that when you eat an actual cherry your taste buds are so knocked out of whack by the extra-strong chemical flavors that you can't even appreciate the vibrant, fresh, luscious flavors your mouth is encountering.

When you remove Frankenfoods from your diet, something magical happens. After a few days, your taste buds return. Suddenly you understand what a carrot tastes like. What an apple tastes like. What a mango tastes like. What sweet is really supposed to taste like.

If you stick with the program for 22 days, you will enjoy powerful results. The weight will come off. The joy in your life will increase. As your new habits start to settle in, you will feel better and better—and learn that you actually *like* eating vegetables and fruits on a regular basis.

You will feel amazing, and you will begin to crave those fresh, delicious foods.

The foods that comprise a balanced plant-based diet may be entirely new to you, or part of your current way of eating, but rest assured that by the time you reach day 22, these will be the mainstays of your delicious and rejuvenating diet.

- **Plant protein:** There are a ton of different types of protein sources for plant-based diets, from kidney beans and lentils to lesser-known options such as spinach and sweet potatoes.
- **Nuts and seeds:** Full of healthy fats and protein, these are where you can find great snacks as well as additions to salads and side dishes. Try flaxseeds, chia, almonds (and almond milk), as well as pumpkin and sunflower seeds.
- **Green veggies:** This is the source of all sorts of healthy vitamins and minerals, as well as fiber. Dark, leafy greens are a priority, but that doesn't mean you can't add in some colorful purple kale or mix it up once in a while.
- **Fruits and other veggies:** Satisfy your sweet tooth with mangoes, bananas, and pears, but also with bright veggies like bell peppers and beets. The more colors, the better.
- **Healthy starches:** Not all starches are bad; you just have to be conscious of your choices and eat starches that offer a lot of nutrition, such as sweet potatoes, squash, whole-grain and brown rice, quinoa, and steel-cut oats.

The goal of the 22-Day Revolution plan is to get you back to eating the bounty that nature has provided you: all of those savory and spicy veggies, sweet fruit, chewy and crispy grains, in their most natural state possible. With my simple and delicious recipes, you don't need a live-in chef to eat like you've got one. (Although meals delivered to your door can help: see 22daysnutrition.com for resources.)

If you eat plants and move away from processed, unhealthy foods, you will go a long way toward improving the quality of your life and losing any extra weight. It's true! Many of the diseases plaguing us, from diabetes to high blood pressure, heart attacks to obesity to acne, are the product of dietary indiscretion and sedentary lifestyles. What happens when you make the shift to eating real, plant-based foods, like cauliflower and apples and broccoli and oranges and raspberries and quinoa and black beans and basil?

You completely revolutionize your life and your health.

4

YOUR FOOD = YOUR HEALTH

MARLIS IS A BEAUTIFUL, ACTIVE woman who was in her sixties when I met her. She had been slim in her youth, but as she got older, ten and then twenty extra pounds crept on, which she attributed to age. She wasn't necessarily overweight, but she'd been feeling sluggish and tired. Marlis was inspired to try the 22-Day Revolution after spending a vacation with her son, who had tried the program and loved it, and was still living plant-based. Since she loved cooking, she really enjoyed preparing and tasting new dishes, and quickly fell in love with the feeling she got from eating clean, organic, cruelty-free food. Her energy went through the roof, she lost the stubborn weight she had assumed was a natural side effect of aging, and she found that she was sleeping better than she had in decades.

As she completed the 22-day program, Marlis realized that before, she had not given much thought into what she was putting into her body: where it came from or how it was grown. She was thrilled with the feeling of abundant energy, better sleep, and improved mood she was experiencing, and she felt proud of the choices she was making.

She stayed with her son for a month, and when she went back home, she continued her new lifestyle, which was already feeling like second nature. A short while later she was due for her annual checkup, including routine blood work.

Her doctor asked her to come back in to go over her results. That was certainly unusual, and she began to worry. They only called you when something was wrong, right? And when they asked you to come in, something must be really wrong.

She walked into her doctor's office with much trepidation and took a seat, ready for the worst.

"What have you been doing differently?" her physician asked her.

Maris said, "I went on a vacation, and my son was on this new diet, so I tried it, and I really like it. I eat plant-based now."

And her doctor said, "Whatever you're doing, don't stop! Your results came back better than they have in years!"

Marlis was thrilled to learn that her cholesterol levels had lowered, her fasting insulin levels were lower, and while she was never overweight, she also lost a few unwanted pounds. She was grateful that she had discovered the plant-based lifestyle, and even prouder of the fact that she took the initiative to explore.

I've always said that our health is the one area of our lives we can't delegate or leave up to someone else to care for. Your thoughts, actions, and daily habits have the power to rob you of your health and make you gain weight, or keep you slim, healthy, and vital.

EATING FOR HEALTH AND VITALITY

If you found out that something you've been doing unconsciously for your entire life has been hurting you, wouldn't you want to stop? How about if what you were doing unconsciously was the reason that you were heavy, tired, and sick? Of course you would. Who wants to weigh fifty or even ten pounds more than they should? Who wants to miss out on the joys of life because you have to go to the doctor, or worse, the hospital? Nobody!

So here are the facts: If you are overweight and/or obese, if you feel fatigued all the time, if you have prediabetes or diabetes or heart disease, if you have stomachaches, heartburn, a bloated belly, acne . . . the source is likely to be your food. All that stuff you consume that comes in plastic wrappers in bright fluorescent colors is responsible for your feeling fat, tired, and sick. All the processed animal products and dairy products and sugar products that you think you crave are actually hurting you!

So what are you going to do about it?

If you are ready to start eating food that makes you healthier, stronger, leaner, and happier, you are holding the map to your health in your hand. Because food can be the greatest source of our health, and eating plants means giving yourself the best health possible. By eliminating animal products like meats, dairy, and eggs, and eating a diet based on plants, fruits, vegetables, and grains, we can reverse the trend and make ourselves healthier instead of sicker, stronger instead of weaker.

PLANT-BASED EATING IS JUST BETTER FOR YOU

The most nutritious, best diets for our bodies consist of live foods from the earth. Scientific research has shown that vegans and vegetarians who eat a plant-based diet have lower rates of cancers, stroke, and heart disease (which is still the number one killer in the United States). Vegans are thinner. Vegans are healthier. Vegans live longer. The benefits of a plant-based diet cannot be overstated.

Just as being fit and empowered can stem from your meals, so can being overweight, or experiencing high cholesterol levels, high blood pressure, diabetes, or asthma. Change your food and you change your symptoms! Eating fruits and vegetables has been proven to lower cholesterol levels, decrease blood pressure, prevent and even reverse diabetes, decrease asthma attacks, and increase the body's metabolism, helping you to burn calories more efficiently.

If you want to lose weight and keep it off, plant-based eating is the best way to go about it. Plants have fewer calories, more fiber, and less unhealthy fat per ounce than meat. Instead of one average fast-food meal you can have a huge salad with hummus, beans, shredded veggies, and vinaigrette dressing, and about six cups of fruit for dessert. That's a lot more food than you would eat at one meal, so you can see how filling up on a plant-based diet gives you more nutrition with a lot fewer calories. That's why I teach my clients to balance their training with their nutrition—because plants plus exercise is a winning combination.

Even if you aren't yet in the habit of fitness, just eating plants can help you lose weight. According to Dr. Neal Barnard, a plant-based diet increases the body's metabolism, burning calories up to 16 percent faster than the body would on a meat-based diet. And according to research done at the Loma Linda University School of Public Health, vegans are, on average, 30 pounds lighter than meat eaters. That's the value of eating plants.

The fact is that if you eat a well-balanced diet founded on plants and you are active throughout your day, you can lose the weight you want to lose. Even if you don't have a trainer or a gym membership, you can do it. A 2006 report suggested that losing weight as a vegetarian is not dependent on exercise. How is that possible? Vegan food is stored and burned in a different process than nonvegan foods. A plant-based diet helps your body *burn more calories after meals*, while meat and processed foods are stored as fat, causing fewer calories to be burned.[11] You can be extremely healthy with a sensible diet as long as you are generally active—even if you don't go to the gym twice a day.

The best thing you can do for yourself is active training with a healthy diet. What you want to avoid is active training with a poor diet. As we saw with my first spin clients back in Miami, if you do a lot of spinning or running or resistance training, and you follow that up with the kinds of meat- and grease-laden foods they serve in strip malls and food courts and the convenience store, you will never lose weight or feel your best. For one, you're probably taking in more calories than you are burning, and thus not ever losing the weight. And two, you're taxing your body and causing inflammation when you work out—but you don't give your body the foods it needs to replenish. So you're doing double damage.

Eating a well-balanced plant-based diet, full of mangoes and grapefruits and melons and millet and black beans and kale and peppers and all the other delicious plants out there, is the way to get the right amount of calories and help your body reduce inflammation—exactly what you need to feel your best.

PLANTS, NOT PILLS!

If you are worrying about your health, I'd like you to take a moment to think about how your concerns are probably a lot like your neighbors',

---

[11] S. E. Berkow and N. Barnard, "Vegetarian Diets and Weight Status." *Nutr Rev.* Apr 2006; 64 (4):175–88. DOI: http://dx.doi.org/10.1111/j.1753-4887.2006.tb00200.x [PubMed].

and your neighbors' neighbors. All the way down the street, across your town or city, and throughout your state and the entire country, people are suffering from poor health because of the food they eat. The problem is personal to everyone who has buildup in their arteries and excess fat around their waists and their livers, and to each physician who has to explain to their patients that their health is seriously at risk. It is also a problem that is of national concern.

Our country is getting sicker and fatter, while health care costs just keep rising and rising. Heart disease is the leading cause of death in the United States, followed by cancer.[12] Doesn't that make *not* getting sick in the first place the soundest possible plan?

That's what the Finnish government decided in the 1970s, when doctors realized that the population was dying of preventable diseases at very young ages.[13] Young men were dying of heart attacks! Over a period of around ten years, measures were rolled out to change the way people ate: to decrease the amount of animal-based saturated fat (like butter) and to increase the amount of fresh produce they consumed. By 1995, mortality from heart disease among 30-to-64-year-old males was reduced across Finland by 65 percent.

But here in the United States, where we are so proud of our lifestyles and our achievements, we keep eating food that we already know threatens our health and longevity in very real and serious ways. And despite all the research about how important it is to eat plants, there's a lot of pressure to keep eating junk. In 2012, fast-food restaurants spent $4.6 billion advertising their food products to kids. That's a lot of effort to convince us to keep feeding ourselves the processed junk foods that are making us sick![14]

A study of half a million people between the ages of 50 and 71 determined that those who ate the most red meat also had the highest BMIs, exercised the least, and ate the fewest fruits and vegetables. Among those who ate the most red meat and the most processed meat, there was increased risk that they would die of cancer or cardiovascular

---

[12] http://journals.lww.com/journalpatientsafety/Fulltext/2013/09000/A_New,_Evidence_based_Estimate_of_Patient_Harms.2.aspx, accessed November 21, 2014.

[13] http://www.who.int/chp/about/integrated_cd/index2.html, accessed June 25, 2014.

[14] http://www.fastfoodmarketing.org/fast_food_facts_in_brief.aspx, accessed August 18, 2014.

disease.[15] According to the Dietary Guidelines Advisory Committee, plant-based diets are associated with a reduced risk of cardiovascular disease and mortality.[16]

A report published in 2013 in the *Permanente Journal* exhorted doctors to advise their patients to eat plants. According to the report, eating plants is an inexpensive, cost-effective way for people to get better instead of sicker. They defined healthy eating as a plant-based diet: "a regimen that encourages whole, plant-based foods and discourages meats, dairy products, and eggs as well as all refined and processed foods."

The study goes on to say that eating plants instead of processed foods may lower body mass index, blood pressure, and cholesterol levels. Plus, patients who start eating plants may need less medication. This is incredible news for people worrying about diabetes, blood pressure, and heart disease.

A plant-based diet can help to repair your body after years of damage from eating meat and processed foods. Food really is your best medicine.

Here's how plants can help:

Obesity. Researchers have demonstrated that there is a positive association between obesity and eating meat.[17] In 2006, a review of 87 published studies found that eating a vegan or vegetarian diet helps people lose weight. They also reported that vegetarian populations have lower rates of heart disease, high blood pressure, diabetes, and obesity.[18]

---

[15] R. Sinha et al., "Meat Intake and Mortality: A Prospective Study of Over Half a Million People." *Arch Intern Med.* March 23, 2009; 169 (6): 562–71. DOI: http://dx.doi.org/10.1001/archinternmed.2009.6. [PMC free article] [PubMed].

[16] Report of the Dietary Guidelines Advisory Committee on the Dietary Guidelines for Americans, 2010: to the Secretary of Agriculture and the Secretary of Health and Human Services. Washington, DC: Agriculture Research Service, U.S. Department of Agriculture, U.S. Department of Health and Human Services, May 2010.

[17] Y. Wang and M. A. Beydoun, "Meat Consumption Is Associated with Obesity and Central Obesity Among U.S. Adults." *Int J Obes* (Lond) Jun 2009; 33 (6): 621–8. DOI: http://dx.doi.org/10.1038/ijo.2009.45. [PMC free article] [PubMed].

[18] S. E. Berkow and N. Barnard, "Vegetarian Diets and Weight Status." *Nutr Rev.* April 2006; 64 (4):175–88. DOI: http://dx.doi.org/10.1111/j.1753-4887.2006.tb00200.x. [PubMed].

Diabetes. Do you want to improve insulin sensitivity and decrease insulin resistance? Eat plants. In a clinical trial of people with type 2 diabetes, 43 percent of subjects on a low-fat vegan diet improved insulin sensitivity and decreased insulin resistance.[19] Another study showed that vegetarians have approximately half the risk of developing diabetes as nonvegetarians.[20]

High blood pressure. In another report, from 2010, the Dietary Guidelines Advisory Committee advised the U.S. departments of Agriculture and Health and Human Services that vegetarian diets were associated with lower systolic blood pressure and lower diastolic blood pressure.[21]

Heart disease. Plants are an effective treatment for coronary heart disease, too. One of the biggest names in heart disease treatment is Dr. Dean Ornish, who believes that lifestyle changes—including the adoption of a plant-based diet—can have a positive impact on wellness. The Lifestyle Heart Trial studied the effects of intensive lifestyle changes on atherosclerosis. Ornish's plant-based eating regimen suggested that fat make up 10 percent of calories, protein make up 15 percent to 20 percent, and carbohydrates make up 70 to 75 percent. Cholesterol was restricted to five milligrams per day. After just one year, 82 percent of the patients who had been diagnosed with heart disease and then followed his program had some level of regression of atherosclerosis afterward. Meanwhile, more than half the patients in the control group—who *did not* follow the plant-based diet—had their atherosclerosis get

[19] N. D. Barnard et al., "A Low-Fat Vegan Diet Improves Glycemic Control and Cardiovascular Risk Factors in a Randomized Clinical Trial in Individuals with Type 2 Diabetes." *Diabetes Care.* August 29, 2006 (8): 1777–83. DOI: http://dx.doi.org/10.2337/dc06-0606. [PubMed].

[20] A. Vang et al., "Meats, Processed Meats, Obesity, Weight Gain and Occurrence of Diabetes Among Adults: Findings from Adventist Health Studies." *Ann Nutr Metab.* 2008; 52 (2): 96–104. DOI: http://dx.doi.org/10.1159/000121365 [PubMed].

[21] Report of the Dietary Guidelines Advisory Committee on the Dietary Guidelines for Americans, 2010: to the Secretary of Agriculture and the Secretary of Health and Human Services. Washington, DC: Agriculture Research Service, U.S. Department of Agriculture, U.S. Department of Health and Human Services, May 2010.

worse.[22] After five years, the group who followed the plan experienced improvements similar to results from patients who had taken medication.[23]

Eat plants! Lower blood pressure, fewer incidences of diabetes, regression of atherosclerosis . . . the evidence is clear that plants are the right choice for all people, especially those who are ill.[24] If the food you eat is making you sick, eating plants can be as beneficial as taking medicine. Why rely on prescriptions when you can enjoy platefuls of gorgeous greens and grains and get similar benefits?

Embrace the power of plants over pills!

ANIMAL, MINERAL, VEGETABLE

You don't need to eat animals in order to get all of your vitamins and minerals. This is a common misconception, especially from people who have not had a lot of exposure to hale and healthy vegans and vegetarians. I get questions about getting enough protein, enough iron, enough calcium—and I'm pleased to let you know that you will get all the nutrition you need on a plant-based diet (except for vitamin B_{12}, as you'll learn below).

Think about it: Where did all the nutrition in the animals you have been eating come from? Plants! Plants are the original source of all minerals in the animals that you have been consuming. Studies have shown that in a comparison of vegetarians to nonvegetarians, the vegetarians were eating *more* magnesium, potassium, iron, thiamin, riboflavin, folate, and vitamins, and *less* total fat.

[22] D. Ornish et al., "Can Lifestyle Changes Reverse Coronary Heart Disease? The Lifestyle Heart Trial." *Lancet.* July 21, 1990; 336 (8708): 129–33. DOI: http://dx.doi.org/10.1016/0140-6736(90)91656-U [PubMed].

[23] D. Ornish et al., "Intensive Lifestyle Changes for Reversal of Coronary Heart Disease." *JAMA.* December 16, 1998; 280 (23): 2001–7. DOI: http://dx.doi.org/10.1001/jama.280.23.2001 [PubMed].

[24] "Nutritional Update for Physicians: Plant-Based Diets." *Perm J.* Spring 2013; 17 (2): 61–66.

The vitamins and minerals in your food are all important players in your body's health. As you'll see below, micronutrients are integral for the health of your skin, your organs, your blood, your bones, and your muscles. Nutrient-rich vegetarian meals will make you leaner and, in the long run, healthier.[25] At the same time, the key is eating *well-balanced* meals. Eating a variety of fruits and vegetables is the best way to make sure you are getting all of your energy nutrients, your minerals, and your vitamins A, the Bs, and C. It's also a great way to make sure you're getting all the fat, carbohydrates, and protein your body needs.

KEEP THE BENEFITS! STICKING TO THE 22-DAY REVOLUTION PROGRAM HELPS YOU . . .

Fight diabetes. Roughly 370 million people are living with diabetes, and according to the International Diabetes Federation, that number is expected to soar to upward of 550 million by 2030. Type 2 diabetes is entirely preventable, and plenty of research suggests that a plant-based diet can help ward off the disease.

Lower your blood pressure. Lots of research, including from the Harvard School of Public Health, suggests that a diet loaded with fruits and veggies can help control hypertension. About one in three American adults suffers from high blood pressure, meaning they're at higher risk for heart disease and stroke— two leading causes of death in the United States.[26]

Keep your heart healthy. Harvard researchers tracked the health habits of about 110,000 people for 14 years, and found that the higher folks' intakes of fruits and vegetables, the lower their chances of developing cardiovascular disease. Specifically,

---

[25] B. Farmer et al., "A Vegetarian Dietary Pattern as a Nutrient-Dense Approach to Weight Management: An Analysis of the National Health and Nutrition Examination Survey, 1999–2004." *J Am Diet Assoc.* June 2011; 111 (6): 819–27. DOI: http://dx.doi.org/10.1016/j.jada.2011.03.012 [PubMed].

[26] http://health.usnews.com/best-diet/best-heart-healthy-diets, accessed November 21, 2014

people who averaged eight-plus servings of fruits and veggies a day were 30 percent less likely to have a heart attack or stroke, compared to those who had fewer than 1.5 daily servings.

Lose weight. There's plenty of research suggesting that vegetarians tend to consume fewer calories, and thus weigh less and have lower body mass indexes than nonvegetarians. Opting for fruits, veggies, and whole grains in lieu of meat will likely leave you feeling fuller on fewer calories.

Get plenty of fiber. Fiber keeps you "regular" by aiding in digestion and preventing constipation. Plus, it may also lower cholesterol and blood sugar levels. Following a plant-based diet means chowing down on loads of fruits and veggies, which are packed with fiber. Just one cup of raspberries or cooked green peas amounts to eight grams of fiber or more, according to the Mayo Clinic.

See clearly. As you may know, the vitamin A in carrots aids night vision. Your eyes might also thank you for a plant-based diet rich in spinach, kale, corn, squash, kiwi, and grapes. The lutein and zeaxanthin pigments in these foods are thought to help prevent cataracts and macular degeneration.

PLANTS, FOR THE BEST OF YOUR LIFE

I'd like you to make the rest of your life the *best* of your life.

Whenever anybody comes to me with a story about wanting to reverse heart disease or diabetes, or to lose ten or twenty or fifty pounds, inevitably I learn about something deeper . . . a difficult relationship with food, or a parent whose bad habits rubbed off a little too well, feelings of insecurity at work or in relationships. I hear about illness and loneliness and uncertainty and depression.

What I tell them is that our mental and emotional well-being have so much to do with what we eat. The powerful nutrition found in plants can help alleviate depression! When you are unhealthy, when you feel unwell or heavy or unattractive or lethargic, everything about life feels harder. Difficult situations can feel overwhelming or insurmountable.

We have less kindness or compassion for everyone, from the stranger driving too slowly in front of us to our friend who always manages to say the wrong thing. Depression and mood swings have been linked to poor nutrition, while eating plants and getting all those vitamins and minerals can ultimately help you emotionally and provide an overall sense of well-being and positivity.[27]

The effects of eating a plant-based diet are beneficial for health and wellness—and that includes every area of your life. When you feel great, and when your body is buzzing with the energy and nutrition from a plant-based diet, everything is easier. Developing the habit of eating plants gives you the energy to deal with life—the energy to live your life in a positive, kind, and compassionate way, and to make the right choices for yourself, so you can be your healthiest, inside and out.

<hr />

[27] http://www.webmd.com/depression/guide/diet-recovery, accessed August 18, 2014.

PART TWO

GET READY, GET SET:

Setting Yourself Up for Success

5

DAILY STRATEGIES FOR SUCCESS

THERE'S A FUNNY LITTLE PLAQUE that I've seen in Cuban restaurants. Just a little saying: *Hoy no se fia, mañana sí*—"We don't do credit today; we'll do credit tomorrow." And of course, what it means is that they'll *never* do credit. How many diets have you started "tomorrow"? How many unpleasant tasks around the house will you get to tomorrow? But really, tomorrow never comes.

If you really want to change, you have to be ready to start *today*. The 22-Day Revolution has become a national challenge and movement, but it is more than that: It is your personal challenge and your personal revolution. When it begins is up to you. How long the benefits last is up to you. If you want to make a real change, and you want to make that change permanently, you can. You can transform—you just have to *begin*.

STICK TO THE RECOMMENDED PORTIONS

During the first two weeks especially, it is very important to stick to the recommended portions. When you switch to a plant-based diet, you'll be consuming fewer calories, because the foods are less calorically dense. As you embark on this program, you'll need to break your bad

PORTION SIZES:	
Beans and legumes	½–1 cup
Grains, like rice, quinoa, millet, oatmeal	½–1 cup
Vegetables	1–2 cups (if you're really hungry, add another cup of plainly prepared veggies)
Fruit	1 cup
Fats like avocado	½ cup
Nuts, raw and unsalted, seeds	¼ cup
Olive oil	1 tbsp.
Vinegar/lemon/lime for dressings	to taste, as desired
Nut butter	1–2 tbsp.

habits of overeating and overindulging. It may be uncomfortable and you may feel hungry at times, but that's okay. Your body is adjusting to the correct portion sizes and will soon thrive without the stress of digesting too much food.

At the end of your 22 days, your body will have adjusted to the recommended portion sizes and you'll be able to eat intuitively without overdoing it. The goal is to develop health habits and to understand restraint.

If you're trying to lose weight, stick to the lower number within the ranges above. If you're embarking on the program for its myriad health benefits, then feel free to enjoy the upper end of the range.

If you're not seeing the results you hoped for, be sure to check your portion size. That is the number one reason progress falters.

Recently I saw this happen firsthand when I was helping out the sister of a friend of mine. He had great success with the 22-Day Revolution—and became a permanent soldier, transforming his own health and his family's—and wanted to get his sister, Alison, involved in the plant-based party. He kept after her for two years before she finally agreed, and when she did, she totally went for it. She filled her kitchen with fruits and vegetables and whole grains, and changed the way she ate.

When he called her a week later to see how it was going, she hadn't lost a pound. How was this possible? He got me on the case. Since I had known her for years, I went over to her house to see what the story was. She invited me to stay for lunch, and I agreed, because I was hungry and I thought it would be a great opportunity to see for myself how she used the program. Alison had prepared a delicious quinoa-based salad, full of vegetables and herbs and greens, and I was thrilled to see how this woman, who would have typically made herself a bologna sandwich on white bread with bright yellow mustard, had already evolved.

But as I watched, Alison ate one portion, and then two, and then three. Right away I understood how she had derailed herself. She was eating the right food at the right time with the right mind-set. But she was eating *too much*. She wasn't paying attention to her portions. And she hadn't yet gotten to a point where she could sense that subtle moment when her body was full and it was time to put down that fork.

Once we identified the issue and she learned to manage her portions, the weight started coming off.

If you've gotten used to eating too much, the journey toward eating the right amount of food might feel like being hungry to you. As long as you are eating three well-balanced, 80-10-10 meals a day (remember, that's 80% carbohydrates, 10% protein and 10% fat), you're getting the proper nutrition you need and providing plenty of fuel for your body.

You'll see encouragement to eat mindfully and thoughtfully throughout this book, as well as reminders to eat with restraint. Being mindful helps you enjoy your food, and so does eating with restraint. If you want to avoid stomachaches and bloating, if you want to lose weight, eat slowly and enjoy each bite; then stop when you have consumed your portion. And remember that it takes twenty minutes for your body to give the signal that you're full. With time, your body will thrive from getting just enough food and not having to digest too much. The hunger pangs will go away, and you'll soon discover the feeling of being comfortably satisfied. At this point in your journey, you'll be ready to learn to eat according to how you feel.

At the beginning, don't worry about feeling hungry! Exercise restraint to set healthy new habits and to achieve the best weight-loss results.

Recently, I had a call from a friend who wanted to do the plan, a man in his sixties who had finally had his wake-up call. He had a distressing conversation with his physician, who had convinced him that if he didn't stop eating red meat and rich desserts, he was going to have a heart attack.

"I've got to do this program," he said. "I really want to do this."

I was so happy! This was a dear friend, and for many years I had been after him to make a change, and finally he was ready.

I sent him the plan.

He called me back right away and said, "Well, what happens if I get hungry?"

I said, "Then you know you're doing everything just right."

He said, "What? What's that supposed to mean?"

I explained that the reason he was never hungry now was because he was overeating.

"That's why you weigh three hundred and ten pounds," I said gently. "In order for you to get healthy, there are going be a few windows you have to walk by, thinking, 'I wish I could.'"

He finally understood that he had to embrace the feeling of hunger. At first he felt anxious when he would feel the first pang of an empty stomach. But he was able to get used to it slowly, and begin to eat to the feeling of satisfaction, not fullness. He has lost more than eighty pounds and no longer considers himself a candidate for a heart attack as he once did. He feels and looks better than he has in decades.

SNACKS

Within the next 22 days, you can eat one snack every other day at most, as needed. Remember, you're trying to get used to eating just three meals, and as your body adjusts, you may need a snack to tide you over. And there's room for dessert! Enjoy two desserts from the recipe section during your 22-day program.

Suggested snacks:

- Nuts, raw and unsalted (remember the portion size: ¼ cup)
- A piece of fruit
- Cut veggies with 2 tbsp. hummus
- 1 tbsp. of nut butter with celery, apples, pears
- Half serving of a smoothie (recipes in chapter 17)

NO IDLE SNACKING

During weeks one and two, you're going to be getting used to being conscious of your habits and learning how it feels to eat a plant-based diet. It's important to commit to three meals a day—and just as important to commit to being mindful of what happens between those meals.

Marie was in her twenties, and had been struggling with her weight since she was a teenager. She decided to try plant-based for the first time after reading about the success so many had experienced with it. Marie was extremely committed to going 100 percent plant-based, but the results weren't there for her in the first few days, and it took about a week for her to realize that her challenge wasn't sticking to plants; it was changing her eating habits.

You see, Marie was a big snacker. When she embarked on the challenge she just swapped out the snacks she was eating for "plant-based" snacks, though she wasn't eating plants, but processed foods that used to be plants.

As you'll see on your menus, when I say "snack," I mean a piece of fruit that is so clearly a fruit that a toddler could identify it. Just because sugar is vegan does not mean that it belongs in your food! When you eat plant-based snacks, eat fruits and veggies, not chips, crackers, pretzels, or cookies.

Marie got to work on figuring out the mechanism for her snack habits. It wasn't long before she realized she had developed a friendship with food that was self-destructive. She turned to food (more specifically her snacks) anytime she needed to vent, celebrate, think, relax—well, just about anytime she had a feeling . . . hence why she always came up empty (food doesn't solve any problems, but rather complicates them with additional feelings of failure). The minute she figured out that her snack habit was keeping her from her goals, she worked on replacing bad habits with healthier ones (in her case eating veggie sticks for the crunch factor, because she was a big chip lover, or distracting herself with a walk or just a quick call with a loved one), and success began to follow.

Marie lost 15 pounds during her 22-day program. She continued to eat a plant-based diet after completion and she has lost 47 pounds to date. Today Marie is in control of her health and happiness, and has also added a few habits, like surfing and running, which make her smile.

NO ALCOHOL FOR 22 DAYS

I'm going to keep this one short and sweet: For the course of the 22-Day Revolution, please avoid alcohol. I'll tell you three reasons why: 1) you are drinking your calories; 2) alcohol leads to dehydration, which makes you hungrier and can lower your willpower, leading to bad food decisions; and 3) your palate will start to crave old habits. Later on, after your three weeks, once your habits have shifted and you have begun to experience the benefits of plant-based eating, you can decide for yourself how to make the occasional glass of beer, wine, or liquor a part of your new healthy lifestyle.

I realized just how important being aware of alcohol consumption can be during an experience with another eye-opening testimonial from a good friend and client, Beth. She was forty pounds overweight and—as she professes—constantly on yo-yo diets. She willingly tried eating plant-based and appreciated how many great foods she could have while significantly improving her health, but could never make it to 22 days. Her willpower would crumble and she would slip back into old patterns before reaching her goal. Ultimately, she thought this program was not for her.

I wanted to learn more, so I asked her to give me examples of her daily meals. Everything checked out from Monday to Thursday afternoon, but that was where the journal ended. When I asked about what she eats on the weekends, she said, "Well, I still eat vegan, but I have to have my vodka, which is low in calories and sugar compared to other drinks." I had to smile, because Beth prides herself on being the master of redirection, and here she was doing it to me. I said, "I didn't ask what you drink; I asked about what you eat." She couldn't help but laugh and said, "When I drink, I start out eating consciously, but then I find myself eating chips, fries, and all the things I deprived myself of . . . well, because it's the weekend—and it's still 'vegan'!"

The problem with Beth wasn't just that she was drinking her calories—which is one of her issues—but that it was leading to old eating habits and binge eating. Worse, the next day she woke up with the right attitude, but by the afternoon the cravings were creeping into her palate and mind. She started with a compromise—"I'll have one vodka and club soda—'hair of the dog'—and no appetizer, just a vegetable crudité." One drink would inevitably lead to three drinks, and before she knew it, she was back on her drinking-and-bingeing cycle for the entire weekend. By Sunday, she felt this program was not for her.

I finally convinced Beth that her health was worth a 22-day shot, and that I was confident she could do it. She broke through the first week, her hardest, and felt a new level of clarity and energy on the second week. By the third week she was empowered, inspired, and unstoppable. Beth continued with the program and lost 45 pounds in five months. Today she monitors her drinking and is in control of her diet.

Beth is the first to say that if she can do it, anyone can. As for me, I just want people to try it for 22 days and let the program accomplish the rest.

USE YOUR SCALE

Recently, I asked a client how much he weighed. He said, "I haven't gotten on the scale since you left. I never weigh myself. I have scale phobia!" He wasn't joking. He was scared of the scale. But of course, it wasn't the scale he was afraid of; it was a fear of failure. But without checking in, how can you win?

The scale is your friend, so I invite you to weigh yourself first thing every morning. Once you're on the program, the scale keeps you in balance. If you think that you're eating right and you get on the scale, and tomorrow you weigh one pound more than you weighed today, you can say, "Whoa, wait a minute; I can fix that." Getting on the scale every day helps you keep yourself in check! When you weigh yourself, you're getting an objective view of your progress. It's not personal. It's just math, and it keeps you aware.

Unconscious eating is like using a credit card. On a daily basis, you aren't aware of the sum total of your actions. You aren't counting every dollar—you aren't conscious. But at the end of the month, the bill comes and your jaw drops open. "Who spent all this?" Well, you did. By the time the bank starts sending you letters in the mail—return, nonsufficient funds, return, nonsufficient funds, return, nonsufficient funds—you're way past the point where you can turn back easily.

If you don't use a scale regularly, it's the same thing. You go to the doctor once a year and you get on the scale and he says to you, "You gained twenty pounds." Next year, another 20. That's how weight comes on. No one goes from 120 to 320 pounds overnight! They go 120, 122, 125, 126, 127, 130, 134, 136, 138—and if you're not paying attention, it keeps creeping up. That's how you gain weight. It's math! It's hard to refute the scale. Twenty extra pounds, year after year, puts you in a position where you have to work that much harder to get back to a healthy weight. And it's much easier to keep up than it is to catch up. It's a lot easier to stop the action the day after than it is three months after.

If you get on the scale and you've gained a pound or two or three, analyze your day. Reflect on yesterday. The scale teaches you to be consciously aware of what you are doing.

It tells you that it is time to go through your mental checklist:

- Did I eat to 80 percent fullness at every meal?
- Did I walk away from every meal feeling overly full?
- Was I drinking my calories?
- Was my sleep right?
- Did I exercise yesterday?
- How many meals did I have and what did I eat?
- Did I graze?
- Did I have a few too many vegan desserts?
- Was I eating vegan Frankenfood, or was I really eating plant-based food?
- Did I eat too much salt? Am I retaining water?
- And for women: Am I getting my period?

The scale is a tool for health. It's like when the doctor listens to your heartbeat or tests your blood sugar. It's simply a measure. You have to know how you're doing in case you need to tweak something! If you see the number go up instead of down, you get the opportunity take a closer look at your habits.

FOCUS ON YOUR MOTIVATION

Why do you want to transform? Your reasons for getting healthy are important to your success. Your motivation is what will keep you on track when temptations call to you. It is what will tell you to go work out instead of sleeping in for another half hour. It is what will sway your hand toward the carrot sticks and celery instead of the potato chips. Your motivation matters in the real world!

Some people want to get skinny. The problem with chasing skinniness is that it's a temporary fix; it's a Band-Aid approach to a problem that's much deeper than just being skinny. If you set out to lose weight for an upcoming event, say a wedding, when it's over, what happens? You balloon back up again, because the motivator was temporary and not sustainable. If you think of wanting to see your son or your daughter walk down the aisle in twenty years, that is long-term, and much more sustainable.

Perhaps you're beginning this program because you've had a troubling conversation with a doctor. I'm so happy you've decided to take charge of your health—but motivation brought on by fear doesn't last long, either! One good visit to the doctor and it's back to the old habits. Ultimately, the fear of dying is not sustainable. Instead, consider the reasons to live—and not just to live, but to live well—for your family, your kids, your spouse, your significant other, your brother or sisters, siblings, parents, grandparents, extended family members, friends. For you. For the beautiful world that we live in. To be able to travel. To be able to enjoy those wonderful moments in your life.

More than being thin, more than living forever, the desire to live well and keep loving the people we love *is* sustainable. That is what makes you get up in the morning and want to work. Right? That's what makes you have a smile on your face and put your best foot forward. If you focus on the right motivation, it becomes easier to make this lifestyle sustainable, easier to create a system that is sustainable, easier to create habits that are sustainable, and easier to create a lifestyle that is conducive to how you want to feel.

THE PILLARS OF SUCCESS

Ultimate success comes from a combination of different factors that all impact one another. If you want to flourish, if you want to enjoy your whole, happiest life, there are five pillars of success.

Pillar 1: Diet. Proper diet and the benefits of nutrition are something you should know a lot about if you've read part one of this book. If you want to be healthy, you have to pay attention to your food. You have to eat plants!

Pillar 2: Exercise. The benefits of exercise complement a healthy diet, and by combining the two, you'll be supporting all your good work and strengthening your heart, lungs, muscles, and bones.

Pillar 3: Sleep. If you want the nutrition you give your body to be able to help heal and repair your muscles and organs after you work out, you're going to need rest. Adequate sleep is fundamental for good health; it helps you regenerate and release stress. It's also fundamental for feeling energized during the day. People who don't sleep enough make poor choices, are more irritable, and snack more.

Pillar 4: Stress management. Stress takes a terrible toll on your body, your work, and your relationships. If you don't take care of the first three pillars, your energy levels dip and your stress levels rise. There are many aspects of life that can raise our stress levels: issues at work, problems with relationships, hard news about your health or the health of someone you love. Eating well, getting enough exercise, and getting enough sleep are all great ways to manage your stress.

Pillar 5: Love. Having plentiful love in your life is also a pillar of your success. Human beings are not built to survive alone! We are social beings who thrive with companionship, friendship, family, and pets. Which brings us to a very important part of being successful at anything you do: your support systems. Your parents and children and sisters and brothers. Your friends. The people who care about you. The pets that show you unconditional love. The healthier you are, the more readily you can take care of them—and the easier it is for them to support you, and the more enjoyable everything becomes! Nobody wants to be a burden on their family. Keeping ourselves healthy is paramount if we want our loved ones to be able to support us in joyous ways instead of difficult ways: as we grow and change for the better. As we go to school and graduate. As we have children and build families. As we run marathons and host parties to celebrate our achievements.

Treat yourself with love and kindness and watch yourself flourish!

HOW TO START RIGHT NOW

Where are you right now? What time is it? If you're feeling inspired, like you'd like to start your 22 days, I'd like to point something out: You can actually start right now. You don't have to wait for tomorrow. The clean slate starts here, at this moment, no matter where you are, no matter what the clock says. If it's nine a.m. and your kitchen has no healthy foods. If it's noon and you are in the local airport. If it is three p.m. and you are taking a quick pause at work. If it's Sunday evening and you are about to join your friends for dinner at your local favorite restaurant. You can still start *now*.

1. **Take a deep breath.** Make a conscious decision to set yourself up for success. Then take action.

2. **Clean up your kitchen.** If you've got the time to tackle it immediately, head into the kitchen and start making a difference. On page 88, you'll find specific directives for how to accomplish this as painlessly as possible.

3. **Go shopping for fresh foods.** You can skip immediately to the day-one menu on page 110 and go buy the foods *today* that you need to start living a brand-new life. In fact, I encourage it. Then, over the course of the next days and weeks, you can continue to read and learn about how it all works and how you can make the most of your experience.

4. Call the restaurant. If you already have lunch or dinner plans, you can still start right now. Plant-based eaters go to restaurants! They go to parties! If you have a reservation for your next meal and you want to start today, just look the menu up online and make a plan. Since you aren't going to eat what you usually eat, and you don't need to make a big deal of it to your friends, you can just decide in advance what you'll order. You don't need to be challenged; you just need to be ready. Find the menu. Read it. If you'd like, call ahead and say, "Hey, I'm a vegan. I'm looking for options. I'm looking for healthy, clean food." (Check out our guide to eating in restaurants on page 212.) You can also eat a handful of raw almonds before you go to the restaurant or event to make sure willpower is on your side.

5. Sleep on the wrong side of the bed. I'd like you to wake up tomorrow with a sense that something is new and changed. You're going to do this by changing how you sleep tonight. So sleep on the other side of the bed, or spend the night in the guest bedroom. I want you to wake up tomorrow with a fresh view, with the feeling that something is different.

You're about to set out on a path of habit change and life change, so I'd like you wake up on day one with a new view, and the awareness that something has changed.

And on day 22, you will see that the "something" that has changed is *you*.

6

THE 22-DAY REVOLUTION
NUTRITION PRIMER

AS YOU SHOP AND COOK your way through the
menus, you'll be getting a healthy ratio of fats, carbohydrates, and
protein with every dish, along with vitamins, minerals, and phytonutrients.

A well-balanced meal contains:

80 percent carbohydrates
10 percent protein
10 percent fats

Let's look at some specifics.

COMPLEX CARBOHYDRATES

There is a very common misconception that carbohydrates are bad for
you. There are different types of carbohydrates—simple and complex—
that can have drastically different impacts on your diet and health.
Simple carbohydrates are made up of one or two sugar molecules and
are the quickest form of energy, and very rapidly digested. When choosing between simple carbohydrates it's best to go with those found in

foods such as fruits and vegetables which are full of vitamins, minerals and fiber while avoiding them in the form of sweets, candy, soda, processed and refined sugars which are void of vitamins, minerals and fiber. These processed and refined sugars are often referred to as "empty calories" because they have little to no nutritional value. Complex carbohydrates have three or more sugars strung in long complex chains (hence the name) and are high in vitamins and minerals, often rich in fiber, and slower to digest, which is how they provide sustained energy. Complex carbohydrates are found in foods such as whole grains, vegetables and legumes. When we consume carbohydrates, our bodies react in one of two ways: We burn them for energy, or we convert them to fat which are stored in fat cells. Can you guess which one happens most often? Once the sugar is released into our digestive tract, the pancreas detects it and releases insulin to deal with it. Insulin helps regulate the sugar level in our blood (the more sugar, the more insulin is released). Insulin helps store all of the excess sugar in the liver and muscle tissue as glycogen and in fat cells. Sometimes our body struggles with putting away too much sugar too quickly, and too much insulin is released, which ultimately causes our blood sugar to drop . . . *bonk!*

Imagine you're packing for a trip. You take out your suitcase. If you dump all your clothes in at once, creating a jumbled, creased mess, the suitcase will be overstuffed. If you take each item of clothing and place it, folded, into the suitcase, everything will fit and remain organized.

Much like the methodical packing of your suitcase, after you eat complex carbohydrates with fiber, your body can effectively handle the storage of energy, and your energy levels stay balanced all day. On the other hand, just like dumping your belongings into the suitcase, simple carbohydrates digest quickly, leading to a surge of sugar in your bloodstream, a chaotic situation that isn't resolved easily. Often your body overreacts by releasing too much insulin to process and store the sugar, leaving you in a sugar crash. And then you crave more sugar, and the vicious cycle begins.

We need carbohydrates because they are the body's main source of fuel (all the tissues and cells in our body use carbohydrates for energy), but we need the right ones (fruits, vegetables, whole grains, legumes) for balanced energy levels and optimum health. Carbohydrates have gotten a bad rap in trendy diets over the last decade, but we should be focusing on the source and type of carbohydrates we eat.

Vegetables and fruits offer healthy amounts of high-fiber complex carbohydrates, exactly what your body needs. Carbohydrates are broken down by your body into their smallest components, glucose, which is essential if you want energy for all of your physical functions. Your brain, nervous system, and entire body rely on the carbohydrates you eat! Every move you make, every thought you think is powered by the complex carbohydrates in the fruits, vegetables, grains, and legumes you eat. The issues that you hear about when people complain about "carbs" arises from situations where real food is replaced by processed carbohydrates full of added sugars, like cupcakes and pizza. Avoid over-processed carbohydrates; eat complex carbohydrates (such as vegetables, whole grains and beans) and you will be full of energy all day long!

PROTEIN

Every cell in your body uses protein. Protein is made up of amino acids, which your body uses for everything from building muscle to creating hormones and enzymes to growing your hair and nails.[28] Your DNA is like a program that tells the amino acids how to group together to perform whatever function your body needs. Each one of your genes has instructions on how to build a protein molecule out of amino acids.

Some amino acids, the ones that cannot be made by your body but are crucial for your health, are called essential amino acids, and they come from your food. You can get amino acids from eating plants, meat, eggs, or dairy. Meat contains the full array of essential amino acids, because it is made of muscle tissue, which is one of the things your body uses all that protein to build.

The beauty of eating a variety of plants is that you will get the full array of essential amino acids. Some plant-based foods offer all the amino acids you need; complete protein sources include quinoa, chia, hempseed and buckwheat. Combining grains and legumes, like rice and beans, is another way to ensure that you're getting all of your aminos. That's why variety matters here!

When shifting to a plant-based diet, some of my clients have expressed concern that they might not be getting the protein they need if

[28] http://www.webmd.com/men/features/benefits-protein, accessed August 19, 2014.

GRAINS

Amaranth, cooked
1 cup,
9g protein

Brown rice, cooked
1 cup,
5g protein

Buckwheat
½ cup dry,
12g protein

Millet, cooked
1 cup,
8g protein

Oats
½ cup dry,
6g protein

Quinoa, cooked
1 cup,
8g protein

BEANS

Black beans, cooked
1 cup,
15g protein

Chickpeas, cooked
1 cup,
15g protein

Edamame
1 cup,
17g protein

Kidney beans, cooked
1 cup,
16g protein

Lentils, cooked
1 cup,
18g protein

Tofu
½ cup,
10g protein

NUTS

Almond butter
2 tablespoons,
8g protein

Almonds
1 ounce,
6g protein

Cashews
1 ounce,
5g protein

Peanut butter
2 tablespoons,
8g protein

Peanuts
1 ounce,
7g protein

Pistachios
1 ounce,
6g protein

Walnuts
1 ounce,
4g protein

SEEDS

Flax seeds

1 tablespoon, 2g protein

Hemp seeds

2 tablespoons, 7g protein

Pumpkin seeds

½ cup, 6g protein

Sesame seeds

2 tablespoons, 3g protein

Sunflower seeds

½ cup, 15g protein

VEGETABLES

Asparagus, cooked

1 cup, 4g protein

Beets, cooked

1 cup, 3g protein

Broccoli, cooked

1 cup, 4g protein

Green peas, cooked

½ cup, 4g protein

Portabello mushrooms, cooked

1 cup, 5g protein

Spinach, cooked

1 cup, 5g protein

FRUITS

Avocado (Florida)

1 cup, 5g protein

Blackberries

1 cup, 2g protein

Coconut, dried and unsweetened

1 ounce, 2g protein

Dates, medjool

½ cup, 2g protein

Dried fruit (raisins)

¼ cup, 1g protein

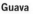
Guava

1 cup, 4g protein

Orange

1 large, 2g protein

Watermelon

1 cup, 1g protein

they only eat plants. In fact, the opposite is true! While plants give you enough protein, many Americans who eat a meat-based diet are eating twice as much protein as they need. Extra protein can't help you build more muscles, and it won't make you stronger.[29] A diet that is too high in protein can lead to diseases like osteoporosis, kidney disease, and some cancers.[30]

The CDC recommends that between 10 and 35 percent of your daily calories come from protein (if you're pregnant, breast-feeding, or an athlete, your requirements will be different). All plant-based foods have varying amounts of protein, and therefore getting enough protein is not an issue on a plant-based diet.[31] A plant-based diet that is well balanced will give your body all the protein you need to thrive. (Check out chapter 14, "Revolution Fitness," on page 217 for more information on how amazing plant-based protein is for athletes.)

FATTY ACIDS

While protein is broken down into amino acids, fats are broken down by the body into fatty acids. Fatty acids are major sources of human energy. You either consume them directly in the form of fat, or some of the carbohydrates you eat are converted into fatty acids and stored in your adipose tissue so that you can have the energy to conquer your daily life with gusto and attack your workouts, especially the moves recommended in chapter 14![32]

Just as essential amino acids are needed by our bodies but not made in our bodies—and so must be eaten by us in our food—there are essential fatty acids that we have to eat if we want to stay fit and healthy. These are omega-3 (divided into two major types: ALA found in vegetable oils, flaxseed and walnuts and EPA & DHA found in seaweed) and

[29] http://www.webmd.com/diet/healthy-kitchen-11/how-much-protein, accessed August 19, 2014.

[30] http://www.pcrm.org/health/diets/vsk/vegetarian-starter-kit-protein, accessed June 24, 2014.

[31] http://www.cdc.gov/nutrition/everyone/basics/protein.html, accessed October 13, 2014.

[32] http://library.med.utah.edu/NetBiochem/FattyAcids/faq.html#q1, accessed June 20, 2014.

omega 6 found in plant oils, walnuts, sunflower seeds, pine nuts. For healthy nails, hair, and skin, among other things, we have to consume our omega-3 and omega-6.[33]

A well-balanced vegan diet includes sources of omega-3s, like ground flaxseed, flax oil, walnuts, and canola oil.[34]

VITAMINS

As you've learned by now, the benefits of a vegan diet are tremendous. Overall, vegans average fewer nutrient deficiencies than average omnivores while maintaining a lower body weight without necessarily losing muscle mass. But there are important nutritional considerations. There are two vitamins that may be difficult to achieve the RDA for on a plant-based diet: vitamins D and B_{12}. As a result, I recommend that you supplement your plant-based diet with these two important vitamins along with a multivitamin: Vitamin B_{12}, and Vitamin D. For a full list of key vitamins and how to incorporate them into your diet, see the appendix at the end of the book.

Vitamin B_{12} is readily available in meat and eggs and dairy but very limited in plants (found in nutritional yeast and some plant-based foods and cereals are fortified with them), and provides many important functions in the body, including blood formation. Too little B_{12} can be serious and can lead to nerve damage that cannot be reversed. Strict vegans and plant-based eaters who eat no meat, eggs, or dairy should take a vitamin B_{12} supplement. Methylcobalamin is a good source.

Two other key components of a healthy diet, especially for a vegan diet, are calcium and iron.

[33] M. S. Rosell et al., "Long-Chain N-3 Polyunsaturated Fatty Acids in Plasma in British Meat-Eating, Vegetarian, and Vegan Men." *Am J Clin Nutr.* August 2005; 82 (2): 327–34 [PubMed].

[34] B. C. Davis and P. M. Kris-Etherton, "Achieving Optimal Essential Fatty Acid Status in Vegetarians: Current Knowledge and Practical Implications." *Am J Clin Nutr.* September 2003; 78 (3 Suppl): 640S–646S [PubMed].

FOCUS ON CALCIUM

Calcium doesn't just come from dairy—there's no reason you can't get adequate calcium with a plant-based diet that includes a variety of veggies, legumes, nuts, and seeds. Needed for strong bones and healthy teeth, calcium is also important for optimum nerve and muscle function, as well as for normal blood clotting. Don't fall for the rhetoric that vegans don't get enough calcium; all it takes is some planning and knowledge about the vegetarian sources of calcium to ensure optimal health and well-being. If there's any doubt as to whether you're getting enough calcium on a daily basis, talk to your physician and/or look for a plant-based supplement.

With just a few smart choices, you can easily achieve the suggested amount of daily calcium. Foods like mustard and turnip greens, bok choy, and kale are great calcium-rich choices.[35] For example, a salad consisting of two cups of kale, almonds, sunflower seeds, white beans and topped with a tahini dressing can add up to 500 milligrams of calcium. A smoothie with a cup of nondairy milk (almond or other fortified nut milk), almond butter, and spinach will get you another 500 milligrams—more than meeting daily requirements.

Use the chart on the next page to find out just how much calcium your body needs on a daily basis, so you know where to start. Then review the long list of plant-based (and soy-free!) sources to choose from.

---

[35] P. Appleby et al., "Comparative Fracture Risk in Vegetarians and Non-Vegetarians in EPIC-Oxford." *Eur J Clin Nutr.* December 2007; 61 (12): 1400–6. DOI: http://dx.doi.org/10.1038/sj.ejcn.1602659 [PubMed].

TOP SOURCES OF SOY-FREE PLANT-BASED CALCIUM

FOOD TYPE	AMOUNT	mg CALCIUM
Nondairy milk, fortified	1 cup	200–300
Sesame seeds	1 oz.	280
Collard greens, cooked	1 cup	266
Spinach, cooked	1 cup	245
Turnip greens, cooked	1 cup	197
Kale, raw	2 cups	180
Broccoli, cooked	1 cup	180
Chia seeds	1 oz.	177
Bok choy, cooked	1 cup	158
Tahini	2 tbsp.	128
Navy beans, cooked	1 cup	126
Great Northern beans, cooked	1 cup	120
Amaranth	1 cup	116
Mustard greens, cooked	1 cup	104
Kale, cooked	1 cup	94
Almond butter	2 tbsp.	88
Sweet potato, baked	1 cup	76
Almonds, whole	1 oz.	74
Adzuki beans	1 cup	65
Okra, cooked	½ cup	62
Navel orange	1	60
Figs, dried	2	55
Sunflower seeds, raw	1 oz.	50
Dried apricots	½ cup	35

DAILY CALCIUM NEEDS

Kids, Birth–12 Months ▶ 210–270 mg/Day
Women, 19–50, and Men, 19–70 ▶ 1000 mg/day
Kids, Ages 1–8 ▶ 700–1000 mg/day
Women, 51+, and Men, 70+ ▶ 1300 mg/day
Kids, Ages 9–18 ▶ 1300 mg/day[36]

---

[36] Source: USDA.

FOCUS ON IRON

One of the most common yet erroneous arguments against a plant-based diet is whether it provides enough iron. Plants also contain iron that is absorbed along with water through their roots, but plant iron can be more challenging for the human body to absorb.[37] But not to worry! There are plenty of plant-based foods that are readily available to provide iron, from greens to fruits to legumes. All you need to do is discover these sources and ensure that your daily diet includes a mix of iron-rich foods.

A plant-based diet should include foods that are rich in iron, like kidney beans, black beans, soybeans, spinach, raisins, cashews, oatmeal, cabbage, and tomato juice. While vegans who eat no animal products may have lower iron stores than nonvegetarians, according to the American Dietetic Association, anemia caused by iron deficiency is unusual, even among strict vegans.[38]

Additionally, it's important to understand how much iron your body requires in a day. For men this is 8 milligrams, while for women it is 18 milligrams (due to the loss of blood during monthly cycles). For postmenopausal women, the daily amount drops to the same as for men, 8 milligrams per day. Pregnant women require up to 27 milligrams of iron per day—so keep in mind that in this case, unless careful monitoring is made, daily iron supplements may be required or recommended by a physician.

So what are the top sources of soy-free, plant-based iron, and how much iron do they provide?

Check out the list on the next page:

[37] A. Waldmann et al., "Dietary Iron Intake and Iron Status of German Female Vegans: Results of the German Vegan Study." *Ann Nutr Metab.* March–April 2004; 48 (2):103–8. DOI: http://dx.doi.org/10.1159/000077045 [PubMed].

[38] W. J. Craig and A. R. Mangels, "Position of the American Dietetic Association: Vegetarian Diets." *J Am Diet Assoc.* July 2009; 109 (7): 1266–82. DOI: http://dx.doi.org/10.1016/j.jada.2009.05.027 [PubMed].

TOP SOURCES OF SOY-FREE PLANT-BASED IRON

FOOD	IRON	SERVING
Spinach (cooked)	6.4 mg	1 cup
Sun-dried tomatoes	4.9 mg	1 cup
Pumpkin seeds	2.5 mg	1 oz.
Swiss chard (cooked)	4 mg	1 cup
Chickpeas	2.4 mg	½ cup
White beans	3.3 mg	½ cup
Lentils	3.3 mg	½ cup
Dark chocolate (over 70 percent)	3.3 mg	1 oz.
Quinoa	2.8 mg	1 cup
Tahini	2.7 mg	2 tbsp.
Hearts of palm	2.3 mg	½ cup
Spirulina	2 mg	1 tbsp.
Dried apricots	1.8 mg	½ cup
Dried currants and raisins	1.5 mg	½ cup
Almonds	1.3 mg	¼ cup

RECOMMENDED DIETARY ALLOWANCE
WOMEN ▶ 18 mg/day
MEN ▶ 8 mg/day[39]

As you can see, achieving even 18 milligrams per day of iron isn't difficult when you combine plant-based iron sources. A simple salad of spinach, dried currants, almonds, pumpkin seeds, and a few sun-dried tomatoes can easily deliver 10 milligrams of iron, while some quinoa combined with lentils and hearts of palm can provide another 8 milligrams. As you can see, with just two side dishes you've covered your bases for the day—simple as that. Add in a few snacks, plus a nibble of dark chocolate, and you've accomplished your goal of 100 percent plant-based iron intake for the day. Don't let the naysayers get in your way— you can easily get enough iron without meat sources.

[39] Source: USDA.

POWER FOODS

Many of our favorite ingredients for healthy and satisfying meals are among the healthiest and most nutritious foods on earth. Incorporate them into your meals to reap the health benefits they offer. Some of my favorites are outlined below.

Cashews

Light in flavor but heavy in nutritional value, the cashew is a nut that can be added to just about anything. Cashew nuts are really seeds found at the bottom of the cashew tree, which originally grew in the warm, tropical climate of Brazil, and are considered a delicacy there as well as in the Caribbean. Luckily for us, they have found their way into homes and grocery markets around the world.

- **Vitamins and Minerals:** The cashew is a terrific source of trace minerals, including copper, manganese, tryptophan, magnesium, and phosphorus. Just ¼ cup of cashews makes for a great snack and contains 20 to 37 percent of these minerals for a mere 189 calories.
- **Boosts Heart Health:** The high concentration of antioxidants in cashews makes them perfect for improving or maintaining the health of your heart, particularly in women. A study based in the UK recently combined the results of four large studies and found that eating nuts four or more times per week could reduce a person's risk of coronary heart disease by 37 percent. That's huge!
- **More Energy:** The copper content in cashews is a major player in helping to maintain healthy bones and tissues, as well as producing melanin for the skin and hair. By increasing the copper in your diet, you can reduce colon cancer risk and ensure good flexibility in your bones and joints.
- **Good Bones:** Magnesium is a huge factor in the development of healthy bones by providing the bones with structural support as well as helping the body regulate muscle tone. It also acts as

a nerve blocker to prevent excess calcium from activating cells, which in turn keeps nerves, blood vessels, and muscles relaxed. By maintaining healthy magnesium levels along with a good source of calcium, you can ensure healthy blood pressure, reduce muscle spasms, and cut the frequency and severity of migraine headaches.

- **Healthy Weight:** Although the high fat content in nuts tends to turn conscientious eaters away, studies have indicated that people who regularly consume nuts are actually less likely to gain weight than those who rarely eat nuts. So don't be afraid to have a handful of cashews for a snack, buy (or make) cashew butter, or add them to cereals and salads.

Almonds

Almonds are amazing nuts: they are chock-full of nutrition, taste great, and are versatile, so it's easy to add them to your diet. They help with brain function, lower cholesterol levels, and even help you have healthier bones and teeth. Just ¼ cup of almonds gives you 45 percent of your daily value of manganese and vitamin E.

- **Heart and Circulatory Health:** Consuming nuts five times per week can reduce your risk of heart attack by up to 50 percent— that's huge! In addition, the skin of almonds is high in flavonoids, which, combined with vitamin E, helps to protect against damage to the arteries, further reducing the risk of heart disease.
- **Good Fats and Lower Cholesterol:** Almonds are high in fat, but they are good fats, which can actually help aid with weight loss. Consuming nuts two or more times per week can give you a 31 percent higher chance of avoiding weight gain. By lowering blood sugar levels after a meal you can stay full longer. High in monounsaturated fats, almonds help you lower LDL cholesterol levels when they replace saturated fats.
- **Alkalinization and Phosphorus:** Very few proteins help make your body more alkaline (the opposite of acidic), which is vital for immune function, energy, and weight maintenance. Almonds

are the only nut that helps alkalinize your body. They are also a good source of phosphorus, which is a major factor in the development and maintenance of healthy bones and teeth.

Almonds can be found in whole form or slivered, as well as almond meal, almond flour, or almond butter. Besides munching on raw almonds, you can toast them and add them to cereals, salads, and entrees. Natural almond butter can be used to replace peanut butter, while almond meal and flour can be used for baking or in smoothies.

Embrace the healthy benefits of almonds by carrying them with you as a snack and combining them with other healthy nuts, such as cashews and pistachios.

Pumpkin Seeds

Sometimes referred to as "the world's healthiest food," pumpkin seeds offer a variety of minerals, including zinc and manganese. While hulled pumpkin seeds are the easiest to consume, removing the husk can also cut down on vitamin E levels. Whole roasted pumpkin seeds can make for a tasty snack, while raw pumpkin seeds (shelled) can be added to soups, salads, and granolas. You can also buy pumpkin-seed oil to add to soups and smoothies.

So, when you're in need of an uplifting snack, reach for those pumpkin seeds and enjoy some of these health benefits:

- **Lots of Antioxidants:** By now you're probably tired of hearing "it's full of antioxidants" for every health food, but pumpkin seeds lead the pack. What sets pumpkin seeds apart from other foods high in antioxidants is that they offer a wide variety of antioxidants, including a range of forms of vitamin E.
- **Mood Boosting:** Pumpkin seeds are full of L-tryptophan to help boost your mood, as well as provide your body with the long-term energy it needs to get through the day without the two p.m. sugar crash.
- **Reduced Risk of Cancer:** Antioxidants in pumpkin seeds help to reduce oxidative stress on the body, which can cut down on

your risk of certain cancers, including breast and prostate cancer. Pumpkin seeds also contain cucurbitacins, compounds that can kill cancer cells, as well as having antibacterial properties. In postmenopausal women, pumpkin seeds can help reduce the risk of breast cancer.

- **Antimicrobial:** Pumpkin seeds have long been used in alternative medicine (starting with Native Americans) to help fight fungal and viral infections. Most of the antifungal and antimicrobial properties found in pumpkins are due to the presence of chemical compounds known as lignans.

- **High in Vitamin K:** Raw pumpkin seeds are high in vitamin K, which helps blood clots form after tissue damage, for faster healing and to prevent excessive bleeding after injury.

- **Fights Menopausal Symptoms:** That's right, pumpkin seeds have been shown to fight the symptoms of menopause. A 2011 study showed that regular consumption of pumpkin-seed oil can help reduce headaches, joint pain, and hot flashes—as well as helping to balance mood. But that's not the only reason to eat the seeds; the same study found that pumpkin-seed oil also improved good cholesterol levels, and helped to reduce blood pressure.

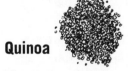

Quinoa

There's a reason quinoa, pronounced "keen-wa," has been making headlines and leading healthy-eating trends. Related to Swiss chard and beets, quinoa is a fantastic food to add to your diet for many reasons. Many people think that quinoa is a grain—like wheat or rice. But really it's a vegetable seed.

- **Excellent Protein.** For vegetarians and vegans, quinoa is an excellent source of protein that contains the nine essential amino acids that your body needs to function optimally. Quinoa contains around 20 percent protein, which is higher than rice, millet, or wheat. Adding quinoa to meals in the form of salads, sides, or main courses can ensure that your body receives adequate protein to build and rebuild tissue.

- **Packed with Riboflavin (B₂) and Magnesium.** Quinoa is an excellent source of riboflavin—which has been shown to help increase energy and reduce the occurrence of migraines, as well as helping cells function optimally. Meanwhile, magnesium helps to prevent hypertension by relaxing the muscles around your blood cells.

- **Low-Calorie.** One quarter-cup of quinoa, uncooked, contains just 172 calories—24 of which come from protein and a mere 12 from sugar. It's also gluten-free. Introducing quinoa to replace other grains, including rice, can help to manage hunger and weight.

- **Low GI and High-Fiber.** Quinoa has a low glycemic index, so it's perfect if you want to maintain your blood-sugar levels for regular energy throughout the day. Compared to popular grains, quinoa has twice as much fiber to keep you full longer, as well as lowering cholesterol.

- **Good Source of Iron, Lysine, and Manganese.** Having the proper balance of iron in your diet helps your muscles function properly to supply oxygen to the brain as well as regulate body temperature and enzymes. By ensuring an adequate intake of lysine, your body can repair tissues quickly. And the antioxidant manganese helps to protect mitochondria and red blood cells from damage.

- **Anti-Inflammatory and Promotes Healthy Bone Growth.** Consumption of quinoa has been shown to have anti-inflammatory effects in animal studies—including a reduction in obesity by lowering levels of fat tissue. By including quinoa in your diet you are also promoting healthy growth of bones by assisting the absorption of calcium and the development of collagen.

Quinoa can be used in bars, to replace oatmeal for breakfast, in salads or granola, in soups, or even in homemade veggie burgers—the possibilities are endless. Quinoa can be found in flour form for pancakes, baking, and other treats.

Gluten-Free Oats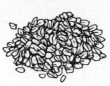

Gluten-free oats make for a healthy snack or meal and offer a ton of health benefits to keep your energy levels up. Check it out:

- **Fuel Your Body:** Oats provide 66 grams of carbs per 100-gram serving, which means you are getting a lot of fuel for your day. Before discounting oats due to the high carb content, consider the dietary fiber they also offer—which helps ensure cardiovascular health.

- **Control Blood Sugar:** Gluten-free oats contain a soluble fiber called beta-glucan, which helps you maintain blood sugar levels by slowing down the body's absorption of sugars while digesting—especially important for avoiding the development or improving the management of type 2 diabetes. Beta-glucan can also boost your immune system by helping it find the source of infection more quickly.

- **Help Your Heart and Circulatory System:** Soluble fiber, found in oats, helps lower total cholesterol levels, leading to a healthier heart and circulatory system. Meanwhile, the antioxidants limit the oxidation of LDL cholesterol, which prevents it from penetrating the blood vessel walls to cut down on plaque buildup. Drinking some orange juice or taking a vitamin C supplement with your oats can help to boost this benefit.

- **Keep You Full:** By slowing digestion and ensuring a regular amount of the appetite-control hormone peptide YY, gluten-free oats can help you feel fuller, longer. Studies have shown that oatmeal is one of the highest-rated foods for satiety—the feeling of being full. If you are looking to start your day with energy and a full feeling to last you until lunch, look no further.

Buying gluten-free oats, as opposed to any other type of oats, ensures that it is easier to digest—particularly if you have a gluten intolerance or allergy. You can find the same varieties of gluten-free oats as regular oats, such as quick oats, rolled oats, or steel-cut oats. Ground oat flour can also be used as a substitute for regular flour in some recipes.

Flaxseed

First cultivated in the Babylonian area around 3000 BC, flaxseed was quickly discovered to be an easy-to-grow, nutritious, grainlike food that packed a powerful nutritional punch. By adding flaxseed to your diet you can feel healthier and help your body fight off disease. Here's what flaxseed can do:

- **Cancer:** Recent studies have indicated that the omega-3 fatty acids found in flaxseed help to reduce tumor occurrence and growth. Additionally, the lignans that occur in flaxseed can help to protect against certain hormone-sensitive cancers without causing interference with drug treatments. The lignans are thought to block the enzymes related to hormone metabolism, which aids in reducing the spread and growth of tumor cells.
- **Heart:** The plant omega-3 fatty acids found in flaxseed are also thought to be great for helping maintain heart health—by lowering blood pressure, reducing and preventing plaque deposits, and helping to treat heart arrhythmia (an irregular heartbeat), as well as reducing cholesterol levels. That's a lot of benefits for one little seed!
- **Diabetes and Inflammation:** There is some information suggesting that lignans may help to improve blood sugar levels, but more research is needed before this can be confirmed. However, there is definite data to indicate that flaxseed can help those suffering from inflammatory illnesses, including asthma, arthritis, and Parkinson's disease.
- **Menopausal Systems:** As little as two tablespoons of flaxseed per day can reduce the hot flashes associated with menopause by as much as 50 percent, and can also reduce the intensity of each episode. Within just one week of adding flaxseed to your diet you can see an improvement, and achieve full benefits in only two weeks.

Besides getting a dose of flaxseed in 22 Days Nutrition Plant Protein Powders, you can add flaxseed to just about any meal. Flaxseed comes as the full seed, or you can get it preground (or grind it yourself) to get the full nutritional benefit. The ground version can be labeled "milled," "ground," or "flax meal," and are all the same.

You can add flaxseed to smoothies, oatmeal, soups, salads, chili, or any other dish. For those who do not eat eggs, you can replace eggs in a recipe by making a "flax egg." Just add 1 tablespoon of ground flaxseed to 3 tablespoons of water, and in a few minutes you'll get a gelatinous mixture similar to an egg. You can also easily incorporate ground flaxseed in baking by taking out an equal portion of flour (up to half a cup per recipe).

Dark Chocolate

If you have to eat any type of chocolate, darker is better. For one, it has less sugar and fat, which is always good for health-conscious eaters. Second, it has higher antioxidant properties, since it contains a higher concentration of cocoa. Dark chocolate also offers the following health benefits:

- **Vitamins and Minerals.** By adding a bit of dark chocolate to your diet, you are giving your body access to trace minerals that are important for optimal function, including potassium, iron, copper, and magnesium. Copper and magnesium are particularly important, as they can assist in preventing type 2 diabetes, as well as help curb high blood pressure and lower the risk of heart disease.
- **Heart Health.** Dark chocolate is excellent for your heart and arteries—just one more reason to make sure you have small regular amounts in your diet. Not only can it lower your blood pressure (don't you feel calmer after some chocolate?), it also may reduce the risk of clots (by preventing platelets from sticking together), and can prevent hardening of the arteries as you age.
- **Better Brain.** By increasing blood flow to key areas of the body, particularly the brain, dark chocolate can ensure optimal bodily function. There are also a few different compounds found in chocolate that help to release endorphins so you feel calm, relaxed, and happy.

- **An Antioxidant Avalanche.** Antioxidant levels are measured by the amount of ORACs (oxygen radical absorbance capacity) contained in the food per 100 grams, and the more, the better. Dry, unsweetened cocoa powder and unsweetened baking chocolate have ORAC values of 50,000 to 55,000, while regular dark chocolate has an ORAC value of 20,000. Those are both much higher than blueberries (9,000) but less than acai berries (102,000). What this means is that a small amount of chocolate contains a high amount of antioxidants, but that doesn't mean you should depend solely on chocolate for your antioxidant needs.

Adding dark chocolate to your diet really shouldn't be a challenge, but it should be done in moderation. Whenever you feel the need for a treat, a small amount of dark chocolate is a good option over high-sugar or high-fat desserts, and can be combined with other healthy ingredients, like fresh or dried fruit.

Remember that not all dark chocolate is the same—look for a high cocoa count to get the most health benefits you can.

GO GREEN

Leafy greens should form the basis of your healthy diet. Every chef around these days seems to love kale, which is amazing, but I'd also like to invite you to look beyond the more familiar greens like spinach to some of their wilder cousins.

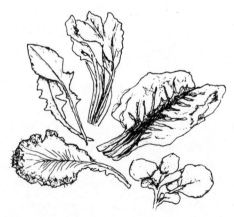

Kale is an excellent green to add to your routine, but it's not the only green that packs a powerful nutrient punch. Rather than boring yourself with the same old salad or cooked greens in your meal, why not try a few alternatives? Mix up your next meal with these delicious greens:

- **Watercress.** An excellent source of antioxidant vitamins (A and C), watercress is also a source of vitamin K for bone health, and contains lutein and zeaxanthin to help protect your vision and support your cardiovascular system. Watercress can be enjoyed cooked or fresh as a replacement for lettuce in salads and anywhere you use greens.

- **Belgian Endive.** Another good source of vitamin A and C, Belgian endive also is a good place to find folate for pregnant mothers, as well as calcium. It is also high in dietary fiber to assist your digestive system and help with weight-management programs by helping you feel full longer. This green can be served raw or cooked; however, it has a slightly bitter taste, so is best when matched with a sweeter fruit or vegetable.

- **Swiss Chard.** A single cup of chopped boiled Swiss chard contains an astounding 636 percent of your daily dose of vitamin K, as well as 60 percent of vitamin A and 42 percent of vitamin C. Swiss chard is also a good source of magnesium, copper, manganese, potassium, vitamin E, iron, and fiber, plus many more. This is one powerhouse veggie!

- **Mustard Greens.** An amazing source of vitamins K, A, and C (as well as copper and manganese), mustard greens can help with cancer prevention and aid the body in removing impurities. To maximize the nutrients in mustard greens, rinse and slice into half-inch ribbons. Toss with lemon juice and let sit for five minutes to activate enzymes prior to cooking.

- **Dandelion Greens.** High in calcium and rich in iron, dandelion greens are an excellent supplement for vegans who want to ensure adequate intake of these nutrients. Dandelion greens are considered a great addition for health-conscious people wishing to detox their system, as they offer excellent liver support and are rich in antioxidants. In the spring you can pick your own greens, or you can find them in many health food stores. Since the greens tend to be bitter, they are best added to smoothies.

■ **Turnip and Beet Greens.** Not only a good source of vitamins K, A, and C, turnip and beet greens are both excellent sources of folate, manganese, and copper. Both greens offer detox support, antioxidant phytonutrients, and anti-inflammatory benefits. The fiber found in beets is considered unique (found only in beets and carrots) and may assist in the prevention of colon cancer. Both turnip and beet greens are excellent served steamed, baked, or in soups and salads.

Changing your selection of greens on a regular basis lets you continue buying local—so you can not only support your local economy but help reduce CO_2 production created during the shipping process. Go, greens!

7

THE 22-DAY REVOLUTION KITCHEN

AT MY HOUSE ON THE weekends, my whole family gets together and comes up with new recipes. Raw, vegan key lime pie? We did it. Walnut tacos? Check. Spanish beans over sweet potatoes? A family favorite. My wife, Marilyn, is an incredible cook, and our boys have developed an appreciation for how good whole-food, plant-based can taste. My family's enthusiasm for discovering new foods to sample and new recipes to try is the foundation for a lot of wonderful things: good health, good habits, and good times together.

We have so much fun! And now you can, too. This chapter is all about setting your kitchen up and preparing to succeed in this new way of eating so you can have maximum fun with the program. We're going to work together to get you into plants so you can get into improved health and better habits. Just like my family did, you can discover the joys of eating plants, beginning with an appreciation for the raw materials: an array of raw fruits and vegetables that will give you all of the nutrition you need to transform your body and your life.

Planning is the key to success—and enjoyment! And what feels better than achieving your goals? The feeling that you get when you cross that finish line is the biggest reward in life. And we all want that feeling! The truth is that nobody ever plans to fail. People just fail to plan. Set yourself up for success by anticipating your needs and making healthy, plant-based food accessible and convenient. Making healthy, life-giving choices at each of your three meals a day is possible—but it requires planning. It requires effort. Cucumbers don't buy themselves and they don't slice themselves!

If you want to step out of the cycle of weight gain and disease and create a new cycle of vitality, planning and following through is the only way to get there. If you were looking for a get-rich-quick scheme, you're in the wrong place. If you're looking for sustainable habits that will give you good health, you're in exactly the right place, because you are about to begin an incredible journey toward health and wellness. You're going to work on seeing which habits are sabotaging you so you can replace them with healthier habits. You're going to see what it feels like to take care of yourself and move toward being the best version of you.

UNPROCESS YOUR PANTRY

There are a number of things you can do to support yourself during the next 22 days. Before plant-based eating becomes a habit, it will take some forethought and some preparation.

Revolutionize your kitchen by cleaning up your kitchen and removing those tempting processed foods that might make habit change more difficult than it has to be. With the right healthy ingredients on hand, the daily menus, and a few simple guidelines, you'll be able to create sustainable habits by putting yourself in a position to succeed.

A 22-Day Revolution kitchen is full of fresh fruits and vegetables and healthy pantry items. It is full of organic produce and organic grains and cereals. It is *not* full of processed foods, sugary foods, lousy-for-your-waistline-and-worse-for-your-heart kinds of food. The more you do to set your home up to support your new habits, the easier you will find it to stick to your intentions. Think about "fast" food. Its biggest selling point is in the name: *fast!* When we aren't used to planning our meals, we wait until we get hungry and then we grab the closest thing. When you are hungry, if healthy food is unavailable and a bag of chips is easy and within reach, all that willpower goes right out the window and you're left with a stomachache and a whole lot of regret.

On the other hand, if you make sure that there are no potato chips, if you make sure that there are sliced carrots and celery and a big bowl of fresh hummus . . . well, then you always have *fast* food that is also *good* food.

I saw the importance of removing processed foods—even if those processed foods are plant-based—from a pantry firsthand while working with one of my clients, Jane, a woman in her fifties, who had been struggling with weight loss since menopause. While in her youth she found it relatively easy to maintain her weight, suddenly the opposite was true: She was gaining weight easily, only to find it nearly impossible to lose. When I met her, she was curious about the benefits of plant-based living, but also sure that it wasn't the kind of thing she would do for very long. Even though she warned me that this "lifestyle" probably wouldn't stick, I was happy to have her get started. The way I see it, once someone experiences the benefits of plant-based living, there's no way she won't be inspired to continue!

Sure enough, Jane lost two pounds on her first day of the challenge and was elated! But then the tides turned, and from day two on, the weight did not move. She even gained a pound back. This was extremely frustrating for her, since she really wanted results.

When she called me to report on her progress and to express her feelings, she blamed the program for her inability to transform, and she blamed her body type. "It just doesn't work for people like me," she said.

I listened carefully, and then we started working to discover what was really going on. I know that plant-based eating works for everybody and every body type, so if it wasn't working for Jane, there had to be an underlying reason. I asked Jane whether she minded going through her days with me so we could figure out what was happening and why her efforts were being derailed.

We went through every day, every meal, and as Jane replayed her days for me, she realized that there were two issues at play: She was consuming too many processed foods, albeit plant-based, and she was eating them in very large quantities.

Just because it is made of plants doesn't mean it isn't processed! When food is processed, the fiber is squeezed out so that you can consume more, more quickly, which means it's easier to overeat. Just because pasta started out as a plant does not mean that if you eat three bowls of it you will lose weight! The opposite is true. And that's what happened with Jane. Once she realized her error and corrected it, she lost the 12 pounds she had been struggling to lose for years.

It is crucial to start with eliminating all of the processed, unhealthy food cluttering up your kitchen. The 22-Day Revolution program is about giving yourself plenty to choose from instead of spending all day trying not to think about what it would be like to indulge in something delicious.

What's in your cupboard right now? Open all the doors and start reading labels.

- **Avoid added sugar.** Added sugar adds calories without any nutrients, and it ruins your taste buds, keeping you from enjoying the full of range of flavors available to you from the natural world. Get rid of sugary drinks, candy, chocolates. Read labels for tomato sauces, salad dressings, peanut butter, pretzels. You'd be surprised what seemingly healthy foods sneak in extra sugar! Natural foods have natural sugar, so instead of focusing on the grams of sugar listed on the label, focus on the ingredients. If "sugar" or "corn syrup" is in there, don't buy it!
- **Lose the artificial sweeteners.** Diet sodas, diet candies, diet anything. Eating plants is about eating natural foods, not artificially created foods.
- **Toss the processed white flour.** Cookies, pancake mixes, cake mixes, white breads, cupcakes . . . get it all out. You don't need processed flours in your meals, because whole-grain flours are versatile and have all the nutrition the grain grew up with, plus the fiber and the bran.
- **Ditch the dairy.** Cheeses, cream, milk. I always tell my friends and clients to avoid milk. There are so many ways to enjoy your food without dairy! Olive oil instead of butter, incredible cashew cheeses, and the best recipe for almond milk (page 250).
- **Free yourself from meat.** Processed meat, deli meat, hot dogs, chicken, fish, seafood . . . Get all of that stuff out of your house and out of your life for good!

Anything that shouldn't be there, bag it up, tie it up, and put it by the door. You can donate it, or if it's really bad for you, you can throw it out. Know that in throwing away this food you're doing something that's going be bigger than you, because you've made a conscious effort to be healthier, to be better, to be smarter, and finally to be a better version of you.

SHOP STRATEGICALLY

The 22-Day Revolution daily menus are packed with all of the goodness your taste buds and your body need to stay happy and healthy. Making good choices at the grocery store will keep you on track for all of your 22-day meals. Shopping strategically is your first defense against common temptations and diet derailments. The more convenient your healthy food is in your kitchen, the more you will reach for it. Your goal is to make fresh fruit and vegetables your closest and most readily available food!

When you fill your cart with fresh herbs, veggies, fruits, and grains, you're getting the ingredients you need to make satisfying, savory meals, and the nutrition your body needs to fight disease and keep you at your healthiest. All of those bananas, carrots, green peas, and strawberries keep your skin smooth, your heart healthy, and your waist trim. As long as you have plant-based foods around you, you'll be armed with exactly what you need to change your habits, change your health, and change your life—over the next 22 days and beyond.

1. **Shop with a list.** For the three weeks of the program, we'll provide a shopping list for every week of the program. You'll find these at the back of the book, along with the recipes.

2. **Shop the perimeter of the store first.** You can hit the internal aisles if you're buying beans or whole grains. But first focus on the perimeter. Fill your cart with all the fruits and vegetables, and then find the other items you need. As you fill your cart, make sure it's a cart you would be proud of if somebody you wanted to impress was looking. (Like an ex. Or your local congressman. Or me.)

3. **Shop after a snack or a meal.** Don't go shopping when you're hungry! Shopping when you're hungry means feeding your eyes, not feeding your body. Have a snack before you go shopping so that you're fully satiated and can make the best choices to fill your kitchen pantry with all of the luscious ingredients you'll love to eat and share all week.

4. **Keep your cupboards full.** Why wait until the cupboards are bare to replenish them? I want you to feel like you have everything you need—and more—during your 22 days.

5. Choose variety. There are so many delicious varieties of familiar fruits and vegetables to look out for! There may be beets swirled red and white, purple daikon, pink sweet potatoes, dark red radicchio, or slender green broccolini, broccoli's tender cousin . . . the more colors you see, the more types you choose, the more you can be sure you're getting all the vitamins and minerals you need to superpower your day. Variety and freshness are what give us the full spectrum of the benefits of all the vitamins and minerals and phytonutrients that we should be getting. And the phytonutrients are part of what make fresh foods taste so good.

NO MORE BULK BUYING

The food you eat comes from somewhere. Have you really thought about its origins? I'm betting that every week or so, you go to the same few shops, hit the same few aisles, and come home with the same products. And most of the food you're buying in large packages has been processed hundreds or thousands of miles away and preserved using chemicals so it can sit on trucks and storage shelves for months until you take it home.

No wonder so many people are unhealthy: because most of us don't really want to deal with shopping (for food, that is), and supermarkets make it easy to go in and out, find what you need under the fluorescent lights, and get home again as quickly as possible, without realizing that it is the choices you make in those aisles that set you up for eating success or failure. If your home were full of bright green broccoli and beautiful red tomatoes and yellow squash that you could easily turn into a healthy meal, you wouldn't need to climb inside a skyscraper-size box of cookies for comfort or "nourishment."

Here's the important point: Bulk buying doesn't work for fresh food (unless you are buying frozen berries for smoothies). Not only doesn't it work for fresh food, but mass purchases of unhealthy processed food are only going to derail your weight loss and goals. Instead of reaching for sugary bars, consider a piece of fruit, or convenient energy and protein bars like 22 Days Nutrition made with whole food ingredients . . . because just like eating healthy, shopping is a habit! So let's replace yesterday's bulk food, processed food, unhealthy food habits with today's revolutionized habit: eating plant-based food.

WHY YOU SHOULD CHOOSE ORGANIC

Organic isn't just a buzzword. The way food is grown impacts our health as much as the way it is prepared. Artificially, chemically, genetically, and synthetically produced foods don't make their way onto our plates only through brightly packaged junk food. When fruits, vegetables, and other plant foods are grown under irresponsible conditions, the quality of our produce suffers, and so do the nutritional benefits. When wax is applied to fruit sold in stores, that apple looks really shiny, but it's also coated in stuff you probably don't want to be eating.

There are over 400 different kinds of pesticides alone used in traditional farming (nonorganic), which requires more energy, more water, and depletes soil fertility. As a result, our bodies are being robbed of the very nutrients we seek for total wellness, needlessly exposed to the dangerous effects of these methods.

Avoiding food high in pesticides can help reduce the risk of certain diseases, including Alzheimer's and Parkinson's disease, autism, and endometriosis. Focus on finding organic, GMO-free produce—so you and your family can enjoy all the benefits of a well-rounded diet, without the drawbacks of residual pesticides.

Eating organic will ensure (as defined by law) that the foods you eat are produced without the use of artificial pesticides and herbicides, growth hormones, genetically modified organisms (GMOs), or synthetic fertilizers. As a result, organic foods can be more nutritious, richer in vitamins and minerals, and higher in nutrient content.

Although pesticide levels are set by the USDA, and fruits and vegetables are typically washed prior to their arrival at your local produce store, many fruits and vegetables can still have residual levels of chemicals. In fact, up to 65 percent of produce can still contain pesticides. But which types of produce are the worst offenders?

Every year, the Environmental Working Group identifies the top twelve foods that have the highest levels of pesticides when they arrive in the store. These are called the "Dirty Dozen."

Here's the breakdown of the 2014 Dirty Dozen:

- Apples
- Strawberries
- Grapes
- Celery
- Peaches
- Spinach

- Sweet bell peppers
- Nectarines
- Cucumbers
- Cherry tomatoes
- Snap peas
- Potatoes

At the top of the list, apples are by far the worst offender—with a whopping 99 percent of conventional apples testing positive for at least some type of pesticide residue. Grapes, a fan favorite with kids, can have up to fifteen types of pesticides on one single grape, something all parents should be aware of. On the far side of the spectrum, many thick-skinned types of produce have lower levels of pesticides, including pineapples, mangoes, and eggplant. Choosing produce lower on the list can be an alternative if pesticide-free produce is not readily available or affordable. If you have to purchase produce from the list, make sure you wash thoroughly before consuming. Removing the peel can also help reduce residual pesticide levels.

Along with fresh fruits and veggies, it's important to consider processed foods made from the produce on the Dirty Dozen list. Apples are used as a base for many types of juice and fruit snacks, so choosing organic versions will help cut down on your and your family's intake of pesticides.

If you can't find organic options in the produce section, check the frozen-food aisle—for example, organic frozen strawberries and peaches are very easy to find.

Plant foods are great—but even greater when they are organically grown, for our sake and the Earth's alike!

MARKET, SUPERMARKET, FARMERS' MARKET, CSA

Where do you buy your produce? If you're ready to try some new flavors and find some fresh favorites, there are loads of ways to do that.

1. **Put the super back into supermarket.** Even if you've been shopping at the same store for years, I'm willing to bet there's a whole array of vegetables and fruits that you haven't

tried—because they're unfamiliar, because you think you won't like them, because you don't know what to do with them. Do yourself a favor and the next time you're at the supermarket, pick up a fruit or a vegetable that you never buy, bring it home, and do some research on what to do with it. Expanding your awareness of the vegetables you can eat and enjoy will help make this journey one that sticks with you on day 23 and beyond.

2. **Find the local farmers' market.** Farmers' markets are all over the place, and they are a wonderful way to explore the seasonal and local offerings where you live. Making a trip to the farmers' market part of your weekly routine is fun for you and fun for your family, and you can all learn and experience together. If you see something unfamiliar at the farmers' market, just ask! Whoever is running the stand will probably have good ideas about how you can enjoy it at home.

3. **Join a CSA.** CSAs are a great way to get involved in local farming. CSA stands for community-supported agriculture (program), and it is a way for you to connect with local growers to get fresh, local goods, all while supporting your community's economy and the livelihoods of one of our most important industries—agriculture. CSAs are big in summertime, because that's when the harvests come in.

CSAS IN DEPTH

Agriculture is a very challenging industry, one where the majority of income is earned during only a few short months. A CSA is a contract between you and a local grower, to provide them with income in exchange for part of their crop. It's the best of both worlds—you get fresh veggies and the grower gets a regular source of income.

How It Works

For an up-front fee, the grower will commit to a weekly delivery of goods (or you can arrange for pickup). Depending on the size of your

investment you may receive a small, medium, or large box of fresh produce per week. You may also be able to customize your box (to a degree)
in order to include or exclude certain veggies.

How is this different from any other "veggie delivery" service? The
key to a CSA is that you are essentially buying a share of the harvest
up-front, rather than just paying for veggies.

Why It's Great

Although some of us could take a trip to the farmers' market on a
weekly basis, for many it's just not feasible. Participation in a CSA gives
you access to fresh veggies for 8 to 10 weeks during the year (or more,
depending on where you live) while you directly support local growers,
with no middlemen. Besides supporting growers, you're also helping the
planet by reducing the carbon emissions, since your veggies are coming
from a much closer location. Additionally, if you can find an organic
CSA participant, then you'll have access to produce free of pesticides
and other harmful chemicals.

Each CSA differs, so find out what's involved prior to commitment.
You may want a CSA that delivers to you, or one that has a nearby
pickup location to make getting your produce easy. In addition, each
farm will also have a different variety of produce offered—find one that
offers a selection you find appealing.

To get started, find out if there are CSAs in your area by looking
online, or check 22daysnutrition.com for more links and information.

THE REST OF THE STORE

Once you've filled your cart with all those abundant fruits and veggies,
then you're ready to hit the aisles.

Canned Food and Beans

These staple items can provide a base for most meals: chili, masala,
soups, curries, sauces, etc. Good items to include are canned and dried
beans, tomato paste and canned tomatoes, vegetable broth, coconut

milk, chili peppers, and pumpkin puree. Look for cans without BPA linings or opt for glass jars.

Seeds and Nuts

Adding seeds and nuts to your meals pumps up your protein and trace minerals, among other nutrients. Some suggestions include chia seeds, flax, walnuts, pumpkin seeds, cashews, and almonds. Nuts and seeds don't stay fresh forever; cycle out your stock regularly, so they don't get stale. Or put them in the fridge once you've opened a new container.

Dried Spices and Herbs

Besides adding flavor to your meal, spices and herbs contain essential micronutrients. Although fresh herbs are best, having a stock of dried herbs on hand can increase the flavor of pretty much any meal, so you can enjoy your vegan dishes, rather than suffering through them. For sweet dishes try cinnamon, ginger, vanilla extract, and even a dash of cayenne pepper. Other suggestions include the standbys thyme, oregano, basil, paprika, cumin, turmeric, and coriander, among others.

Condiments

You can use condiments as dressings, but also as sweeteners, as thickeners, to add flavor, or to create marinades. Some suggestions include agave, almond butter, red curry paste, tahini, coconut aminos, mustard, and nutritional yeast. Some of my favorite dressings are made with a base of tahini and some lemon juice.

Grains

Healthy, whole grains make a great base or side dish and provide protein and carbohydrates. For breakfast, lunch, or dinner, keep the following items on hand: brown rice, quinoa, gluten-free rolled oats, corn tortillas, millet, puffed-rice cereal. For pasta dishes look for healthier options than standard durum semolina—such as quinoa, brown rice, or other gluten-free pasta.

Oils and Vinegars

Much like condiments, oils and vinegars can make a humdrum meal fantastic. Make vinaigrettes or marinades, or use as a healthy base for stir-fry. Suggestions include extra virgin olive oil, coconut oil, balsamic vinegar, and apple cider vinegar—but you can try all sorts of oils and vinegars to add flavor to your meals. (Remember, when it comes to oil, moderation is always important.)

Dried Fruit and Chocolate

Dried fruit is great for everything from salads to desserts, and who can live without a bit of dark chocolate once in a while? You'll find a recipe for Marilyn's mini chocolate-chip muffins in the Revolution Cookbook at the back of the book. Additionally, dates and other dried fruits can be used as sweeteners in smoothies and baked goods instead of sugar.

Beverages

As part of a healthy lifestyle, water is going to be your go-to beverage, but you'll want to have a couple of other liquids on hand. As a base for smoothies or on your cereal, a good-quality almond or other nut milk will work well. And coconut water is a nice addition to smoothies or to help replenish electrolytes after an intense workout.

GET READY FOR SUCCESS!

Are you ready? Then let's go! You've already made the decision to get off the hamster wheel. You've learned about the value of eating plants, and learned how to set your kitchen up to help you create better habits over the next 22 days. You've got a goal, and with the shopping lists and recipes at the back of the book, and the menus in the next section, you've got a plan.

Every time you go shopping, every time you reach into your pantry, be conscious. Be mindful. Don't be habitual! Be a creator of new, conscious habits.

8

THE 22-DAY REVOLUTION
WEEKLY SHOPPING LISTS

GET READY TO GET INTRODUCED to some really delicious fruits and vegetables—or reintroduced to old favorites via some new preparations that will really wow you. The key to healthy plant eating is variety! Before starting this program, you might have been prone to grabbing the same triple-washed spinach in a box every time. Or the same familiar kale. Both of those are wonderful for you, and I love a kale salad—but as you cook your way through the varied and delicious meals in the 22-Day Revolution program, you'll be exposed to new vegetables, grains, and legumes, combined in exciting ways to stimulate your palate.

As you begin to shift your habits and eat your greens and reds and oranges and yellows, you'll start to appreciate the different seasons, so you can have variety at different times of the year. The 22-Day Revolution program is not about deprivation! Deprivation doesn't work and deprivation isn't sustainable. Expand your palate by trying different kinds of squashes, of apples, of berries, of greens, enjoying an abundance of seasonal colors and flavors, along with the health benefits of a fresh, plant-based diet.

■　■　■

ESSENTIAL KITCHEN TOOLS

A Revolution kitchen needs an arsenal:

- Measuring spoons and cups
- Food processor
- Spiralizer (great tool for making veggie pasta)
- Sushi bamboo mat

WEEK 1 SHOPPING LIST

Fresh seasonal fruits and vegetables are the backbone of an exciting vegan diet, but pantry staples round out the fresh produce into a satisfying meal. To prepare for your 22-day program, this week you'll build up your arsenal, stocking up on flours, grains, oils, vinegars, and nuts, as well as all of the fresh fruits and vegetables that you're going to be enjoying.

PANTRY STAPLES:

FLOURS

almond flour

baking soda

brown-rice flour

gluten-free oat flour

tapioca flour

OIL/VINEGAR

apple cider vinegar

balsamic vinegar

coconut aminos

coconut oil

extra virgin olive oil

safflower oil (or canola oil) (high heat)

SPICES/SEASONING

basil leaves (or dried basil flakes)

black ground pepper

cayenne pepper

cinnamon

coriander

cumin

curry

garlic powder

ginger

Madagascar vanilla extract

paprika

parsley flakes (dried)

sea salt

turmeric

CONDIMENTS/MISC.

applesauce

artichoke hearts (1 BPA-free can)

canola mayo

capers

Kalamata olives

maple syrup

nori sheet

pitted dates

vegan chocolate chips

WEEK 1

GRAINS/BEANS/LEGUMES

beluga lentils

black beans

brown rice (short-grain)

chickpeas (1 can of BPA-free)

green lentils

quinoa (actually a seed but usually
    found with grains)

quick oats

vegan and gluten-free bread

PRODUCE

banana

blueberries (fresh)

broccoli

carrots

cauliflower

celery (chopped)

cherry tomatoes (1 small pack)

cucumber (2)

eggplant (1)

fresh fruit (whole)

garlic

Granny Smith apples (3)

grape tomatoes (1 pack)

grapefruit (1)

grapes (green)

Haas avocados (7)

jalapeño pepper

jicama

kale

lemon (6)

lime (3)

onion (2)

oranges (2)

plum tomato (3)

red pepper

romaine lettuce

shallot

spinach

sweet potato (1)

tomatoes (2)

zucchini

SEEDS/NUTS/DRIED FRUIT/NUT MILKS

almond butter or sunflower butter

cashews (raw, unsalted)

chia seeds (2 cups)

flaxseed (milled)

nuts (raw, unsalted)

pine nuts

sesame seeds

tahini

walnuts

almond milk (available plain or vanilla
    flavored. You may want to try both)

coconut milk

WEEK 2 SHOPPING LIST

You've already got a gorgeous stocked pantry full of oils, vinegars, spices, and seasonings that make your veggie dishes sing. This week you'll add to the mix, with some more grains and beans, and a market stand's worth of fruits and veggies. Happy cooking!

GRAINS/BEANS/LEGUMES
black beans
brown rice (short-grain)
lentils (black)
pinto beans (1 BPA-free can)
quinoa

PRODUCE
apple (1)
Asian pears (2)
basil (fresh)
beets (2)
blueberries (frozen)
broccoli
carrots
cauliflower
celery
cherry tomatoes (2 boxes)
cranberries (dried)
cucumber (4)
fennel
fresh fruit
Fuji apple (1)
garlic
ginger
Granny Smith apple (cored)
grapes
Haas avocado (6)
iceberg lettuce
kale
lemon (3)
lime (4)
onion
orange
parsley (fresh)
peppers (2)
romaine lettuce (1 head)
scallion
spinach
sweet onion (1)
sweet potato (1)
tomatoes (8 large ripe)

SEEDS/NUTS
almonds
cashews
sunflower seeds

SPICES/SEASONING
mustard (traditional)

PLUS
almond milk
coconut milk (1 can)
gluten-free oats
hearts of palm (canned)
linguine (gluten-free preferred) (1 box)

WEEK 3 SHOPPING LIST

By now you should be used to picking up your arrowroot flour and your quinoa, and, most important, your cartful of produce. How does it feel to shop consciously, with purpose, and know that you are giving yourself the best of the best? It feels incredible—but you don't need me to tell you that. You already know.

GRAINS/BEANS/LEGUMES
black beans
brown rice
chickpeas (raw in a bag)
chickpeas (1 can of BPA-free)
green lentils
lentils (1 can of BPA-free)
lentils (beluga) (bagged)
quinoa

PRODUCE
alfalfa sprouts (small box)
banana (1 bunch)
basil leaf, chopped (or pinch of dried basil)
broccoli (1 head)
carrots (1 bag)
cauliflower (1 head)
celery (1 bunch)
cherry tomatoes (1 box)
cucumber (6)
eggplant (1–2 large)
fennel
garlic clove
ginger, grated (small bunch)
Granny Smith apples (2)
Haas avocado (7)
jalapeño (2 small)
kale
lemons (3)
limes (6)

onion
parsley
peppers (5 medium, any variety)
pineapple
romaine lettuce
scallions
shallot
spinach (1 bunch)
sweet potato (1 large)
tomato (3 plum)
tomato (8 large)
tomato (cherry) (1 large box)
turmeric
zucchini (1large)

SEEDS/NUTS
cashews (1 cup raw)
flax meal
sunflower butter
walnuts (raw, unsalted)

PLUS
almond milk (vanilla)
applesauce
capers
coconut milk (1 can)
cranberries (dried)
dates
hearts of palm (1 BPA-free can)
hummus
linguine (gluten-free) (1 box)

PART THREE

GO!:

22 Days of Revolution
Meal Plans

9

WEEK 1:
EATING TO BUILD WINNING HABITS

THE BEGINNING OF YOUR JOURNEY! Starting a new way of eating is like going on a trip: You can plan for it, you can imagine it, you can shop for it, but what the experience becomes is something you're going to have to find out for yourself. That's the joy of a personal journey. The way you feel on this program is going to be specific to you. The challenges you face are going to be yours. It is your own inner strength you will have to rely on if your mission is to be successful.

I'm here to tell you that it *can* be successful. You can identify the habits that have prevented you from losing the weight you want to lose, and living the energized, healthy lifestyle you want to live. This is your opportunity to shine a light on those habits, and develop strategies to keep yourself committed to the program. Once you get started, once you begin eating those bountiful foods, it's going to get easier and easier.

And then there's going to be a moment when it gets harder. Because that's life! A diet doesn't happen in a vacuum. Sure, you can go on a retreat for seven days where people prepare food for you, or get picked for a TV show to host you for six months, but at some point you're going to have to go home, where your old habits are waiting for you.

Over the next three weeks, focus your attention on one important lesson every day, using consistent and conscious choices to build new neural pathways to form positive habits. Notice how you feel as you begin eating from the delicious plant-based menu. Soon you'll enjoy the benefits of a full spectrum of vitamins and minerals and you'll feel more energetic, sleep better, and feel a sense of vitality. You are on your way to building the habits that will help you continue on the path to the best version of you.

The 22-Day Revolution program takes planning and cooking. You'll learn the building blocks of a healthy and delicious plant-based diet that will take you well past the 22 days and become staples in your family's repertoire. You should set out to follow the 22-day program closely. I designed the meals to work with one another in providing a balance of macro- and micronutrients. However, I understand that over the course of 22 days, you'll get busy and you'll eat out, and the fundamentals of a demanding life may seep in. I urge you to carve out the time for yourself in this important journey.

But when you can't take the time to cook and enjoy the meal, be prepared. Check out the restaurant's menu online to select a meal that closely replicates the one you're missing. Cook in advance, preparing meals or components of meals over the weekend for a busy Monday. When in doubt, choose a vegetable-based vegan meal, like a salad topped with grilled vegetables and nuts, or a vegetable stir-fry (light oil) over quinoa, or, in a real pinch, create your meal out of several vegetable sides.

I didn't build many repeated meals into the 22-day program, because variety is one of the joys of cooking and eating. But if you find something you love, that's easy to prepare, or that pleases your family, feel free to eat it more often. Try increasing the portions for a dinner recipe, to have enough leftovers for lunch the next day. Make the 22-Day Revolution program work for you. Just be aware of swapping carb-heavy meals including a lot of legumes or grains like quinoa for dinner, as they may curb weight loss.

Remember the importance of the power foods, which form the basis of the meals on the 22-day program. These are among the healthiest and most nutritious foods on earth and you can find them in each recipe by looking for the following symbol: ▲.

Day by day, over the next 22 days, we will slowly instill positive new habits for you to make your own. The new, healthy habits will replace those old ones that have dragged you down, so that afterward, no matter where you are—at home, on vacation, at parties, at restaurants—you'll have the right instincts to make healthy choices!

DAY 1

FEEL POWERFUL

Welcome to day one—the first day of the best of your life. When you woke up this morning, I hope you had the feeling that it was the beginning of something new. The days ahead are going to be exciting and challenging and 100 percent worth the effort. The choices you make, starting today, have the power to change your entire life.

Remember, you don't have to be in great shape to take advantage of the power of working out. Did you know that you burn roughly the same number of calories whether you walk or run a mile? You don't have to go faster. You just have to go.

Make fitness your habit by turning to page 217 for moves you can do anywhere. Or just hit the sidewalk or the road and get your metabolism going. Exercise is the perfect complement to eating plants, because as we've learned, a plant-based diet already turns the temperature up on your metabolism. Getting your fitness in turns that dial another notch. And that's what you want, isn't it? To transform your body. To change your energy level. To build the habits that keep you going strong.

DAY 1 MENU

▶ **Breakfast**

Oatmeal with Banana and Blueberries

Bananas are high-potassium, making them good for your heart, and their sterol content makes them good for your cholesterol levels, and their fiber makes them good for decreasing your risk of heart disease. And bananas are an excellent choice for endurance athletes, with vitamins and minerals, easy to tote and yummy to eat. A 2012 study discovered that consuming half a banana every fifteen minutes gave long-distance cyclists as much energy as sports drinks would have.[40]

INGREDIENTS:

1 cup of almond milk (or other nondairy milk substitute)
½ cup of quick oats (steel-cut oats take a bit longer to cook)
1 banana
½ cup of fresh blueberries

1. Combine oats and almond milk in a pot over high heat.
2. Stir until it comes to a simmer and desired consistency is reached.
3. Pour mixture into a bowl and top with sliced banana and blueberries.

▶ **Lunch**

Quinoa Salad with Lentils

With power foods like quinoa and lentils in one dish, just one serving of this salad gives you plenty of protein, fiber, folate, and iron. Just another reason to enjoy your delicious lunch. . . .

INGREDIENTS:

▲ 1 cup quinoa
  1 cup lentils

---

[40] http://www.whfoods.com/genpage.php?tname=foodspice&dbid=7, accessed July 22, 2014.

½ tsp. fine sea salt

1 tbsp. cumin

1 tbsp. coriander

1 large carrot

dash black ground pepper

handful of spinach

1. Rinse one cup of quinoa in a fine sieve, drain, and transfer to a medium pot.
2. Add 2 cups of water and a pinch of salt. Bring to a boil and simmer until the water is absorbed and quinoa is fluffy (15–20 minutes).
3. Rinse one cup of lentils and transfer into a medium pot.
4. Add 2 cups of water, 1 tbsp. of cumin, 1 tbsp. coriander, 1 large carrot (chopped), 1 dash of black ground pepper
5. Bring to a boil and simmer for 20–30 minutes. Add water as needed to make sure the lentils are just barely covered.
6. Serve quinoa over a bed of spinach and top with lentils.

▶ **Dinner**

Raw Walnut Tacos

TACO MEAT INGREDIENTS:

2 cups walnuts

2 heads of romaine lettuce

1½ tbsp. cumin

1 tbsp. coriander

2 tbsp. balsamic vinegar

1 tbsp. coconut aminos

dash paprika

dash garlic powder

dash black ground pepper

GARNISH INGREDIENTS:

2 Haas avocados

½ pint cherry tomatoes (1 small pack)

½ tbsp. dried parsley flakes

Recipe Continues

pinch black ground pepper

pinch sea salt

1 lime

1. Thoroughly wash and drain the lettuce and tomatoes in a colander or on a paper towel and set aside while preparing remaining ingredients.
2. Combine all taco ingredients in a food processor.
3. Pulse several times until crumbly, making sure not to overblend.
4. Spread the walnut taco meat on the romaine leaves in 4 equal servings.
5. Slice tomatoes in halves.
6. Slice the avocados in half and remove the pit. Peel the skin and cut into small, even pieces.
7. Garnish the walnut taco meat with sliced avocado, tomatoes, parsley, ground pepper, sea salt, and lime juice.

EXERCISE

■ **CARDIO:** Do 30–45 minutes of the cardio of your choice (suggestions outlined on page 222), followed by 10–15 minutes of stretching.

DAY 2

DECIDE THAT YOU'RE WORTH IT

Change isn't easy. As you begin to build the habits that will create the healthy lifestyle that will help you feel and look your best, there are going to be moments when you are tempted to go back to last week's habits. That's when I invite you to remember that you are worth the hard work. You're worth the effort. And you deserve to benefit from the results.

Give yourself the same respect, care, and consideration that you offer to the beings around you. You are precious and valuable. You deserve the best life you can possibly have. So treat yourself well, and feed yourself the best foods available.

When you feel whole and cared for, when you nourish yourself on a daily basis, it shows. And there's nothing more gratifying. There's nothing more empowering. There's nothing sexier.

2

DAY 2 MENU

▶ **Breakfast**

Lean Green Juice

MIX ALL INGREDIENTS IN A BLENDER UNTIL SMOOTH:

4 stalks of kale

1 handful spinach

2 Granny Smith apples (cored)

1 lemon (peeled)

2 pitted dates

1 frozen banana

▶ **Lunch**

Spanish Beans over Sweet Potato

This dish is rich and hearty—and packed full of antioxidants, protein, and fiber. Sweet potatoes originated in South America and were brought back to Europe in the 1500s by Christopher Columbus. Have you ever seen a morning glory, with its brilliant purple flowers in a trumpet shape? Sweet potatoes are a member of the morning glory family,[41] *and just as the flower comes in many shades, so do sweet potatoes. They can be yellow, orange, dark orange, white, and purple. In every case they are sweet, rich, and a yummy base for recipes like my Spanish beans over sweet potatoes. . . .*

INGREDIENTS:

1 sweet potato

1 cup black beans

½ small onion, chopped

1 glove garlic, chopped

1 dash salt

½ tsp. oregano

---

[41] Harold McGee, *On Food and Cooking*, 304.

1 tsp. cumin

1½ tbsp. balsamic vinegar

dash black ground pepper

1. Soak beans overnight. Drain, rinse, and discard water.
2. Place the beans in a medium pot with 4 cups of water, onion, garlic, oregano, and cumin and bring to a boil, then simmer for 45 minutes.
3. Once beans are tender, add vinegar, salt, and ground pepper.
4. Preheat oven to 450 degrees.
5. Scrub sweet potato under running water and dry.
6. Poke a few holes around the potato and place on a sheet of parchment paper.
7. Place sweet potato in the oven for 30 minutes and flip over for another 20 minutes.
8. Remove cooked potato from oven and slice in half after it has cooled a bit.
9. Top with black beans and garnish with tomato and avocado.

▶ **Dinner**

Artichoke, Tomato, and Avocado Salad

Creamy avocados, fresh tomatoes, and the salty brine of the artichokes make this a balanced and satisfying salad. The word tomato comes from the Aztec word for "plump fruit": tomatl. And in fact, tomatoes are a fruit, even though they are widely treated like a vegetable. Tomatoes started out in South America and were domesticated in Mexico; it took a while for them to be accepted in Europe,[42] but once they were, food was never the same again. And they're good for you too, because the salicylates found in tomatoes are beneficial in protecting you against diseases like heart disease and cancer.[43] And the lemony dressing adds healthy benefits as well as a vibrant note. Lemon is a versatile fruit used to treat scurvy, the common cold and flu, and kidney stones, as well as digestion issues,

---

[42] Harold McGee, *On Food and Cooking*, 329.

[43] Ibid. McGee, 256.

pain, and swelling. Researchers think that the antioxidants lemons have, called bioflavonoids, are what make the fruit so good for us.[44] *Lemons (and limes) also contain limonoids, which can fight cancers that occur on the mouth, skin, lung, breast, and colon.*[45]

INGREDIENTS:

1 box grape tomatoes

1 Haas avocado

1 BPA-free can artichoke hearts

1 lemon

2 tbsp. Kalamata olives

dash paprika

1. Into a mixing bowl, slice grape tomatoes into fourths, slice artichoke, peel avocado and chop into equal-size pieces.
2. Add in olives and lemon juice and toss gently.
3. Place into serving bowl and top with paprika.

EXERCISE

RESISTANCE TRAINING: Complete the exercises outlined on page 222.

---

[44] http://www.webmd.com/vitamins-supplements/ingredientmono-545-LEMON.aspx?activeIngredientId=545&activeIngredientName=LEMON, accessed July 23, 2014.

[45] http://www.whfoods.com/genpage.php?tname=foodspice&dbid=27, accessed July 23, 2014.

DAY 3

COMMIT TO THREE MEALS A DAY

Hello, day three. I hope the adrenaline of giving yourself incredible fitness and nutrition this week helped you wake up with a little spring in your step. Avoid the common diet pitfall of grazing, or snacking unconsciously on small amounts, and commit to three meals a day. When you snack, it becomes nearly impossible to really know what you've actually consumed.

I've spoken with so many people who can't understand why they aren't losing weight. They'll say things like, "I usually have an egg white for breakfast and I'll have a salad for lunch. Nine out of ten times I skip dinner." How is that possible? It's possible because they eat all day and they don't remember it. The only meals they are focusing their conscious attention on are the "low-calorie" meals. Once those are consumed, they move through the rest of their days, grazing here and there and never taking a tally, because it's "just one."

As with any new way of eating, there's a learning curve, so be kind to yourself as you adjust to eating just three meals a day, and one snack if you're really hungry.

Want to be successful today and every day that follows? Plan in advance to eat three meals a day.

DAY 3 MENU

▶ **Breakfast**

Chia Pudding (2 servings, so save one for tomorrow!)

INGREDIENTS:

½ cup of chia seeds

2 cups of almond milk

1 tsp. ground cinnamon

1 tsp. Madagascar vanilla extract

1 tbsp. maple syrup

1. Combine all the ingredients in a blender and blend for 1 minute.
2. Place mixture into mason jar(s) with a lid and refrigerate overnight.
3. When ready to serve, stir well and spoon into bowl.
4. Top with fruit and/or seeds/nuts.

▶ **Lunch**

Lentil Soup Garnished with Avocado and Tomato

It doesn't have to be a chilly afternoon to enjoy a warm bowl of this hearty lentil soup . . . and you'll flip when you see how good it is with an avocado garnish!

SOUP INGREDIENTS:

1½ cups dry green lentils

6 cups water

1 tbsp. high-heat safflower oil (or canola oil)

½ onion, finely chopped

¼ tsp. garlic, minced

½ tbsp. cumin

½ tsp. coriander

¼ tsp. turmeric

½ tsp. sea salt

dash cayenne pepper

GARNISH INGREDIENTS:

2 Haas avocados, chopped

3 plum tomatoes, diced

½ lemon, juiced

½ tsp. parsley, minced

dash sea salt

1. In a bowl, mix together all the garnish ingredients and set aside while preparing the lentil soup.
2. Sift through lentils, and rinse well in a colander, making sure to remove any tiny stones that may be mixed in.
3. In a saucepan, heat the safflower oil over medium heat. Add onion, garlic, and a dash of salt, making sure to stir occasionally until onion becomes translucent.
4. Add remaining soup ingredients and bring to a boil.
5. Reduce to a simmer, cover, and cook for about 45 minutes.
6. Stir occasionally to avoid the soup burning or sticking to the pot.
7. Once lentils are soft and tender and desired consistency is reached, serve and garnish.

(about 4 servings)

▶ **Dinner**

Cauliflower Salad

Rich roasted cauliflower paired with pine nuts and grapes makes this salad unexpected—and an unexpected new favorite. Grapes are full of phytonutrients, and research has been done on the benefits of grapes for your cardiovascular health, immune system, and blood sugar regulation, among others.[46]

Recipe Continues

---

[46] http://www.whfoods.com/genpage.php?tname=foodspice&dbid=40, accessed July 24, 2014.

INGREDIENTS:

1 medium head cauliflower

1 lemon (juice)

dash salt

dash pepper

2 tbsp. pine nuts

½ cup grapes (sliced in half)

1. Heat oven to 300 degrees.
2. In a mixing bowl toss the cauliflower with all the ingredients.
3. Place on parchment paper and roast for 15–30 minutes.

EXERCISE

CARDIO: Do 30–45 minutes of the cardio of your choice (suggestions outlined on page 222), followed by 10–15 minutes of stretching.

DAY 4

GIVE YOUR FOOD THE ATTENTION IT DESERVES

Now that you've had several days to get used to eating plants, I invite you to take a closer look at how you eat. What is your habit around eating? Do you eat standing at the counter with one hand in the fridge and the other in your mouth? Do you eat in front of the TV or while reading? Do you eat while you are on the phone? Walking down the street? In your car?

Today, I'd like you to give your food the attention it deserves. You've worked hard to prepare this food, so take some time to really enjoy it. Give yourself space to begin to discover and appreciate the feeling of being satisfied after a meal instead of overstuffed.

Today and every day that follows, see what you can do to get into the moment of food. Sit down when you eat. Eat at a table. Use a real plate and a real napkin. Put on some quiet music. Find a cool, quiet spot to sit and relax in, or find a rowdy bunch of friends to sit with.

The 22-Day Revolution way of eating is not about denying yourself the pleasure of eating—it's about cultivating that pleasure so that your food makes you feel good during your meals as well as after.

4

DAY 4 MENU

▶ **Breakfast**

Chia Pudding

Enjoy the second portion from yesterday!

▶ **Lunch**

Thin-Crust Pizza

Pizza is on the menu in the 22-Day Revolution program! It will satisfy any pizza craving while keeping you on your way to a healthy new you. Make this over the weekend or the night before for a great lunch to bring to work.

INGREDIENTS FOR CRUST:

¾ cup brown-rice flour

½ cup tapioca flour

⅓ cup water

1 tsp. olive oil

½ tsp. sea salt

INGREDIENTS FOR TOPPINGS:

2 medium ripe tomatoes

½ Haas avocado

2 fresh basil leaves, chopped (or 1 tsp. dried basil flakes)

black ground pepper, to taste

INGREDIENTS FOR VEGAN MOZZARELLA CHEESE:

▲ ½ cup raw cashews, soaked

1 cup water

1 tbsp. tapioca flour

1 tsp. lemon juice

1 tsp. apple cider vinegar

½ tsp. sea salt, or to taste

1. To prepare the cheese, add all ingredients into a high-speed blender and blend until creamy. In a saucepan, cook the cheese, stirring often over medium-high heat. Reduce heat and keep stirring to prevent burning. Once consistency has thickened (looks like melted cheese), remove from heat and let cool. Set aside while preparing other ingredients. Leftovers can be stored in fridge up to 5–7 days.
2. Preheat oven to 350. Lightly grease and dust a baking sheet or pizza stone with brown-rice flour.
3. In a mixing bowl, combine the flours with the salt and whisk together.
4. Make a well in the center and add the water and oil and mix with a spoon. If necessary, add 1 tbsp. at a time of water until consistency is reached.
5. Scoop out the dough onto a baking sheet or pizza stone and use hands to shape and press down into desired shape (square/rectangular). Smooth with wet fingers and prebake for about 20–25 minutes.
6. Wash and slice each tomato into 3 thick slices.
7. Remove the pizza crust from the oven and top with the 6 slices of tomato, sliced avocado, cheese (or vegan cheese of choice), and basil.
8. Bake for another 15–20 minutes until slightly crisp.
9. Remove from oven, top with a dash of pepper, slice into 6 square slices, and serve (serves 2)!

► **Dinner**

Raw Zucchini, Carrot, and Cucumber Salad

One bite and you'll agree that zucchini and cucumber belong together. The carrots add a pretty hue, and I just can't get enough of this tahini dressing. . . . And tahini is a good source of calcium.

Recipe Continues

INGREDIENTS:

1 zucchini

1 carrot

1 cucumber

1 tbsp. tahini

3 tbsp. lemon juice

dash sea salt

dash sesame seeds

1. Spiralize the zucchini, carrot, and cucumber.
2. Whisk together tahini, lemon juice, and sea salt.
3. In a mixing bowl, toss spiralized veggies with dressing.
4. Serve and top with sesame seeds.

EXERCISE

RESISTANCE TRAINING: Complete the exercises outlined on page 222.

DAY 5

REDISCOVER WHAT SATISFIED MEANS

■

If you're going to succeed at your revolution, if the foods you are eating now are very different from what you used to eat, there will be a period of adjustment where you get used to what it feels like *not* to be overstuffed. It may feel like hunger, but if you've eaten the correct portion of healthy food, what you are feeling isn't true hunger. It's the feeling of satisfaction.

Restraint is an intrinsic part of enjoyment!

How often do you finish a meal with your gut full to bursting, your pants too tight at the waist, wishing you could take a nap? That feeling of fullness is what makes people gain weight. A feeling of just enough is what you're looking for here.

5

DAY 5 MENU

▶ **Breakfast**

Quinoa Porridge

It's a breakfast that satisfies and gives you the energy to power through your day—exactly what you want out of a breakfast. Get creative and top with different combinations of fresh fruit, seeds, and nuts.

INGREDIENTS:

- ⚘ 1 cup of quinoa
  2 cups of almond milk
  ¼ tsp. Madagascar vanilla
  1 dash of cinnamon
- ⚘ 1 tbsp. milled flaxseed
  1 tsp. maple syrup

1. Combine quinoa, almond milk, cinnamon, and vanilla in a pot.
2. Bring to a boil and reduce to a simmer.
3. Once the quinoa is fluffy, remove from pot, top with milled flaxseed, and drizzle with maple syrup.

▶ **Lunch**

Vegan Sushi Roll

It's a real treat in my house when Marilyn gets the nori sheets and the bamboo mat out. Turning your kitchen into a pop-up sushi bar is even more fun than going out to dinner! (Looks too difficult? It's really not. Stop by your local sushi restaurant, sit at the bar, and order a veggie roll. Once you've seen them make it you'll realize just how easy it is to prepare and perhaps be encouraged to try for yourself.)

This roll can be made with any of your favorite foods. Feel free to substitute any of the vegetables and make it your own. Another vegan sushi roll that is also delicious is made with brown rice, avocado, sliced jicama, spinach, and carrots. Sprinkle with sesame seeds, then cut roll into 6–8 pieces and top each piece with one teaspoon of hummus and one whole salted cashew. The burst of flavor in each bite is so delicious you won't even need soy sauce!

INGREDIENTS:

1 cup short-grain brown rice, cooked

½ Haas avocado, cut in two slices

3 tbsp. raw broccoli, ground in food processor

2 tbsp. raw cauliflower, ground in food processor

▲ 2 tbsp. crushed cashews

1 tbsp. light canola mayo

sprinkle sesame seeds

1 nori sheet

sushi bamboo mat

1. Cover the bamboo mat with plastic wrap.

2. Place the nori with the rough side facing upward.

3. Wet hands and place the brown rice in the middle of the nori. Evenly spread the rice with fingers while pressing down gently.

4. Flip the nori over and place the avocado slices across the middle of the nori, along with the broccoli, cauliflower, mayo, and cashews.

5. Begin to roll the mat, keeping it tight with every move forward, including the sides.

6. Sprinkle sesame seeds and, with a wet knife, cut the roll into 6–8 pieces and enjoy!

▶ **Dinner**

Baked Eggplant with Pico de Gallo

If you like eggplant, you are going to love this dish. The roasted eggplant is the perfect foundation for the creamy, spicy pico de gallo. . . . I'm getting hungry just thinking about it. The flavor comes from roasting the eggplant and adding herbs, onion, garlic. . . . Delicious taste along with health benefits that are out of this world. Parsley has volatile oil components,

Recipe Continues

like myristicin, limonene, eugenol, and alpha-thujene. In studies of animals, myristicin has been shown to inhibit the growth of tumors. Parsley's volatile oils make it a "chemoprotective" food that can help protect us from some forms of carcinogens, like cigarette smoke.[47] Meanwhile, onions help you slow the body's removal of calcium from bones. Eggplant is a great source of phenolic compounds, which function in your body like antioxidants. Eggplant is also good for your heart and protects you against free radicals—and is the most delicious thing you'll ever eat when you prepare my wife Marilyn's Baked Eggplant with Pico de Gallo (available here as well as in my house, when I'm lucky).[48]

INGREDIENTS FOR EGGPLANT:

1 large eggplant

4 tbsp. olive oil (for coating eggplant)

sea salt, to taste

INGREDIENTS FOR PICO DE GALLO:

1 Haas avocado, quartered, pitted, peeled, and chopped

2 medium tomatoes, diced

1 small onion, minced

½ jalapeño pepper, seeded and minced

2 limes, juiced

1 garlic clove, minced

¼ cup parsley, minced (can use cilantro instead)

black ground pepper, to taste

sea salt, to taste

1. Preheat oven to 450.
2. Wash and peel skin of eggplant, then slice into half-inch round slices.
3. Lightly brush each slice with olive oil on both sides and sprinkle with sea salt.
4. Place on a lined baking sheet in the oven for about 8–10 minutes on each side.

[47] http://www.whfoods.com/genpage.php?tname=foodspice&dbid=100, accessed July 24, 2014.

[48] http://www.whfoods.com/genpage.php?dbid=22&tname=foodspice, accessed July 24, 2014.

5. Prepare the pico de gallo by adding all the ingredients in a mixing bowl and lightly tossing together.

6. Once eggplant is cooked, serve and top each slice with pico de gallo and enjoy!

EXERCISE

■ **CARDIO:** Do 30–45 minutes of the cardio of your choice (suggestions outlined on page 222), followed by 10–15 minutes of stretching.

DAY 6

PUT YOURSELF IN SITUATIONS WHERE YOU CAN SUCCEED

If you're like most people, there are some situations that trigger your desires. Who doesn't want candy at the candy shop, cookies at the bakery, sundaes at the ice-cream shop? Sometimes the easiest time to say no is before you walk in the door.

What is your Achilles' heel? Where does your willpower flag? Where does it get really hard to stay strong?

Awareness of what tests us is the first step toward being ready for the challenge. So if you find yourself in a situation that tests your willpower, analyze it and prepare yourself for the next one, because the next situation is coming, and it's coming quickly. If you aren't comfortable yet with saying no, you've got to be careful. Stay away from the doughnut shop! Don't put yourself in a position to be tempted. Don't allow other people's choices to dictate what your day is going to look or feel like.

Use your awareness. Put yourself in situations where you can succeed.

DAY 6 MENU

▶ **Breakfast**

Kale Lean Juice

Kale is a fabulous source of antioxidant vitamins A and C, and apples may reduce risk factors for heart diseases, as well as lower cholesterol, help regulate blood sugar, and control appetite.[49]

MIX ALL INGREDIENTS IN A BLENDER UNTIL SMOOTH:

4 stalks of kale

1 cucumber

1 Granny Smith apple (cored)

1 cup green grapes

▶ **Lunch**

Vegetable Curry

Every bite of this curry is as good for you as it is just plain good—exactly what you deserve at every meal. Broccoli is a power food. It's a great source of protein, dietary fiber, calcium, iron, vitamin C, folate, potassium, and more.[50] *Cauliflower also gives you plenty of the potassium, fiber, and folic acid you need to stay healthy, plus a compound called isothiocyanate that is useful for disease prevention.*[51] *Fresh ginger, veggies, coconut milk: This curry is rich, aromatic, and loaded with health benefits.*

Recipe Continues

---

[49] http://www.webmd.com/heart/news/20110412/apple-good-for-your-heart, accessed July 22, 2014.

[50] http://nutritiondata.self.com/facts/vegetables-and-vegetable-products/2356/2#ixzz 38CMbVECx, accessed July 22, 2014.

[51] http://www.webmd.com/diet/features/cauliflower-health-boost, accessed July 22, 2014.

6

INGREDIENTS:

4 cups mixed veggies (use any mixed veggies of your choice, or try my suggested combination below)

1 cup broccoli

1 cup kale

1 cup peppers

½ cup cauliflower

½ cup spinach

1 onion, finely chopped

2 garlic cloves, chopped

1 tbsp. fresh ginger, grated

2 tsp. curry

dash salt

1 can coconut milk

1. In a large skillet over medium heat, sauté onions, garlic, and ginger in a dime-size dollop of canola oil for 2 minutes.
2. Add in all the other ingredients and bring to a simmer until the sauce thickens and the veggies are tender.

▶ **Dinner**

Beluga Lentil Salad

Tiny black belugas are one beautiful way to explore variety. And in this salad, the dark hue of the lentils gives you extra anthocyanins and really pops against the green and red of the salad.

INGREDIENTS:

1 cup beluga lentils

1 shallot

1 tbsp. lemon juice

1 tsp. apple cider vinegar

1 tsp. sea salt

½ tbsp. coriander

½ tbsp. cumin

1 tbsp. capers

2 tbsp. red pepper, diced

1 handful of fresh greens

1. Rinse the lentils and place them in a pot with 2 cups of water with sea salt, coriander, and cumin. Bring to a boil and simmer until desired tenderness is reached (15–20 minutes).

2. In a mixing bowl, combine the lentils with lemon, vinegar, capers, shallots, and pepper.

3. Arrange lentils over a bed of greens and top with lemon juice and vinegar.

EXERCISE

▨ **RESISTANCE TRAINING:** Complete the exercises outlined on page 222.

DAY 7

MAKE TIME FOR YOU

■

You can't take care of your family and friends, and do your best at work, if you're not taking care of yourself. Stress plays a big part in our overall health and, importantly, in our ability to lose weight and maintain a healthy lifestyle. Making time for yourself, to unwind in whatever way you like, is essential to a healthy and balanced life.

Schedule your free time as you would a dentist's appointment or a conference call. Treat it just like any other appointment and you'll find the people in your life will support you in taking that time for yourself.

DAY 7 MENU

▶ **Breakfast**

Toast with Nut Butter and Blueberries

Just two minutes to make! If you don't have two minutes for the most important meal of the day, then you may want to reconsider how your day begins. A solid, healthy breakfast will get you ready to go! Blueberries are full of anthocyanins that provide good health as well as their deep purple color. They are also a great source of vitamin C, offering nearly a quarter of your daily requirement in just one serving. Vitamin C boosts your immune system, and it also helps your gums stay healthy. If you're looking for fiber, manganese, and antioxidants, eat a cup of blueberries and feel good about your morning.[52]

INGREDIENTS:

  2 slices of vegan and gluten-free bread
  2 tbsp. of almond butter or sunflower butter
  1 banana
  1 cup of blueberries

1. Spread almond or sunflower butter on toasted bread.
2. Top with banana slices and blueberries.

▶ **Lunch**

Chickpea Sandwich

Chickpeas are good for digestion, managing blood sugar, and getting plenty of protein and fiber—and they are also a tasty way to eat your lunch. There's a reason chickpeas are so popular in so many cuisines across the world; just one bite of this chickpea spread should show you why.

Recipe Continues

---

[52] http://www.blueberrycouncil.org/healthy-living/blueberry-nutrition/, accessed July 22, 2014.

INGREDIENTS:

2 slices of vegan, gluten-free bread

1 BPA-free can of chickpeas

¼ cup celery (chopped)

¼ cup carrots (shredded)

2 tbsp. canola mayo

1 tbsp. whole-grain mustard

1 romaine lettuce (head)

1 small tomato

pinch ground pepper

1. Place chickpeas, mayo and mustard in a food processor. Pulse a few times until blended well, but not too smooth.
2. Transfer to a bowl, and mix with the celery and carrots.
3. Place lettuce over toasted bread and top with chickpea spread.
4. Add tomato and a dash of pepper to finish.

▶ **Dinner**

Jicama and Avocado Salad

Crispy, cool jicama; creamy, delicious avocado . . . this is one of my favorites, and we eat it all the time at my house. Jicama is light and crunchy, and a cup contains nearly 6 grams of dietary fiber, about a quarter of your daily dose—good news, since eating fiber can keep you regular and also protect you from hypertension, heart disease, stroke, and obesity.

INGREDIENTS:

2 cups jicama, peeled and diced into cubes

1 Haas avocado

1 carrot (or ½ cup shredded carrots)

⅓ cup diced fresh curly parsley

1 tbsp. extra virgin olive oil

1 lime, juiced

sea salt, to taste

ground black pepper, to taste

1. Wash jicama, carrots, and parsley thoroughly and let dry in a colander.
2. Peel or scrub the carrot, then cut the ends off and slice with a vegetable peeler.
3. Peel and dice the jicama and avocado.
4. Finely dice the parsley.
5. Toss ingredients in a mixing bowl with olive oil, lemon, sea salt, and pepper, and serve.

EXERCISE

▧ **CARDIO:** Do 30–45 minutes of the cardio of your choice (suggestions outlined on page 222), followed by 10–15 minutes of stretching.

10

WEEK 2:
CREATING CONSISTENCY

WELCOME TO WEEK TWO. YOU'VE been eating plants for a week, and you've already faced down some demons and made some connections in your brain related to your new habits—the habits that you are choosing to make you stronger, leaner, and healthier. You've been weighing yourself over the course of the week, and if you've been sticking to the portions, eating three times a day, and exercising, you should have already seen some weight loss.

If you want the pounds to keep coming off, you've got to start week two out strong. You've got to come in determined. Because if you want those benefits to keep piling up, and the weight to keep sliding off, you've got to keep on working the program.

That's why, for week two, we're going to focus on creating consistency. You spent last week building habits around eating plants; you should be feeling great about that! Whenever you have an achievement, it's important to congratulate yourself. The key is *how*. Because sometimes, when we experience some initial success, we start to get a little full of ourselves. We can think, *Oh, look, I've lost eight pounds; surely I can reward myself with a nice cheesecake.*

Stop right there.

If you like the way it feels to lose eight pounds, *keep doing the things that made you lose the weight.* Be consistent.

Because consistency counts. If you've ever met somebody with a skill that absolutely impressed the hell out of you—say a singer, or a dancer, or a mountain climber—you can bet that skill wasn't achieved in a day. Anybody you know who is a professional at anything shows up every day. That's how it works in life. Doing things once, just trying them, doesn't get you results. What gets results is consistency.

If you want to get a degree, you can't just go to school for a week. You have to work hard for four years in order to receive your degree. And then you're still working hard every day to achieve your goal. If you start a business, you have to show up every day. If you get a job, you have to show up every day. Every single day, you have to believe you can do it, and then you have to get out of bed and do it. That's what it takes to succeed. The same is true for your health!

If you want to be healthy, you have to be consistent. You have to work hard. You have to show up every day.

Consistency doesn't say, "I made it, so I can backslide." Consistency says, "I showed up today and I'm doing great, and you know what? I'm going to show up again tomorrow and try a little harder."

Show up every day for the best of your life. Make the most of today and every day. Be consistent!

DAY 8

RUN YOUR OWN RACE AT YOUR OWN PACE

I remember when my sister ran her first half marathon with me. She never thought she could do it. I said, "Trust me. You can do it. You're going to love it."

She told me that she wanted to break two hours, and that was her ultimate goal for the race. I assured her we would, because we had trained with that pace in mind, and we were running her pace.

So we start running. Two miles in, three miles in, four miles in, five miles in. She's feeling good; we're in the groove.

I say, "Jen, we're on target."

"You think?"

I say, "Don't look at your watch; don't worry about it. You're in the right zone; you feel good; you're running your race. Stay with your race."

Then we're at mile ten. Some people are sprinting past us, and Jen gets nervous. Now she's paying attention to someone else's race instead of her own.

So she slows down, because she's discouraged by someone else's success. So I say, "No, don't do that. Run your race. Do what you came to do."

She starts running a little faster.

I say, "Don't speed up; don't slow down. Just stay in your lane."

Now she's looking around; she's saying, "But those guys . . ."

"Jen," I say, "I promise you. I've told you this for a long time, for many, many years. Run your race."

"Okay."

She sticks to her game plan. She runs at the same exact pace we've been running the whole race. We come in just under two hours. Just under. By seconds. Exactly what she wanted to do.

She was so proud! And it all happened because she ran her own race.

That's the message for today. Run your own race. This is your race. Not anybody else's. Just yours. What I've just said is true about a marathon, and it's true for your revolution. It's crucial that you understand it, because it is the difference between success and failure.

Run your own race! No matter what your goal is, other people may be more effective than you. Suzy from the office loses more weight. Or Dan seems to eat whatever he wants and never gains a pound. Forget Dan. Forget Suzy. This is about you.

Run your race. Stay at your pace. You aren't competing with anybody else. And when you get there, as long as you keep going, there is no greater feeling in the world than the day you look at the scale and you look in the mirror and you flex your biceps and you say, "Wow. I did this."

There's something euphoric about going the distance, because you challenge yourself in a way that no one can challenge you. You get to a point where you test your mental fortitude like no else can, with yourself.

And that's where the fun begins.

DAY 8 MENU

▶ **Breakfast**

Immunity Juice

The Baltimore Longitudinal Study of Aging ranked the combination of apples and pears as the second-highest source of flavonols—and that was among all fruits and vegetables. The phytonutrients in pears are antioxidant and anti-inflammatory, and can help decrease the risk of type 2 diabetes, heart disease, and cancer.[53]

MIX ALL INGREDIENTS IN A BLENDER UNTIL SMOOTH:

2 Asian pears

1 Fuji apple

1 cup of frozen blueberries

▶ **Lunch**

Gluten-Free Linguine with Tomato and Basil

Sometimes you just want to settle back with a bowl of pasta . . . and basil just makes it better. Basil, a member of the mint family, has been part of the human diet since the Greeks and the Romans discovered its pleasures (and that is just one of the reasons we think they have such great taste). The basil you will find at the market may have tasting notes of lemon, cinnamon or anise.[54]

Recipe Continues

---

[53] http://www.whfoods.com/genpage.php?tname=foodspice&dbid=28, accessed July 22, 2014.

[54] Harold McGee, *On Food and Cooking.*

INGREDIENTS:

1 box linguine (remember to look for healthier options, such as quinoa, brown rice, or other kind of gluten-free pasta)

4 quarts water

6 large ripe tomatoes

2 tbsp. extra virgin olive oil

1 tbsp. garlic, minced

18 basil leaves

sea salt, to taste

ground black pepper, to taste

1. Heat olive oil and garlic in a large pan with a dash of sea salt over medium-high heat.
2. Wash and lightly chop tomatoes and basil leaves (half the portion) and add to the pan. Let cook for about 5–10 minutes until soft. Set aside to cool.
3. Place tomatoes in a blender (leaving pan aside for later use) and mix until smooth, or when desired consistency is reached.
4. Pour the sauce back into the pan on low heat, and add the remaining basil. Let cook for about 10 minutes, while preparing the pasta.
5. Bring 4 quarts of water to a boil. Add a dash of salt, add the pasta, and stir. Cook for about 6–9 minutes, stirring frequently and making sure not to overcook.
6. Drain and rinse in a colander.
7. Add the pasta to the saucepan and gently toss together.
8. Cover over low heat for a few more minutes, then serve, top with basil, and enjoy. (Serves 4–6.)

▶ **Dinner**

Hearts of Palm Salad

Perfect for picnics or any potluck where you're asked to bring a dish.

INGREDIENTS:

▲ 1 cup quinoa

2 cups water

1 cup hearts of palm, sliced (canned)

½ pint of cherry tomatoes, halved

1 Haas avocado, quartered, peeled, and chopped

1 cup cucumber, chopped

½ cup iceberg lettuce, (or romaine) chopped

⅓ cup broccoli, finely chopped

1 tbsp. extra virgin olive oil, optional

1 lime, juiced

black ground pepper, to taste

sea salt, to taste

1. Rinse one cup of quinoa in a fine sieve, drain, and transfer to a medium pot.
2. Add 2 cups of water and a pinch of salt. Bring to a boil and simmer until the water is absorbed and quinoa is fluffy (15–20 minutes). Makes about 2 cups.
3. In a small bowl, mix together the olive oil, lime juice, pepper, and sea salt.
4. In another bowl, add the hearts of palm, tomatoes, avocado, cucumber, lettuce, and broccoli and lightly toss together with the dressing. Toss in the quinoa once completely cooled and serve.

(Serves 2.)

EXERCISE

■ **RESISTANCE TRAINING:** Complete the exercises outlined on page 222.

DAY 9

UNLOCK YOUR HIDDEN POTENTIAL

■

If you want to achieve success, you've got to commit to the idea that *you can do it*. The potential for success lives inside you, no matter what your experiences or struggles have been until this point.

There's an old story about a farmer who found an eagle's egg, which he brought home and tucked into a chicken coop with all the other eggs. Soon the egg hatched.

The baby eagle was raised alongside the other chicks, and so he did whatever they did, learning with them. Since chickens can only fly for a short distance, the eagle, too, would fly for only short distances. In his mind, he was a chicken, and that was the extent of his natural abilities.

He had no idea that he was an eagle who had the power to soar, so he spent all of his time pecking around in the dirt with the other chickens. One day he saw a majestic bird flying high in the sky, much higher than a chicken could go. He was completely awed!

The hens explained that the bird was an eagle, the king of the birds in the sky.

From his place in the dirt, the young eagle watched the other eagle soar, never realizing that he himself was a king of birds, with the untapped power to soar across the sky.

It's so easy to confuse our view for our possibilities! What you see around you is not an indication of who you are or what your potential is. If you don't like how you feel, change it. Do you set your personal bar based on what you see around you or what has happened in the past—or what you have inside of you? Aim for the sky.

You will never know how much potential you have unless you allow yourself to try.

DAY 9 MENU

▶ **Breakfast**

Homemade Granola with Berries

Homemade granola is so easy to make, and so delicious to eat, that you'll wonder why you ever thought you had to buy it in a store.

INGREDIENTS:

▲ 2 cups of gluten-free oats

¼ cup of maple syrup

▲ ¼ cup (mix) chopped cashews, almonds, and sunflower seeds

½ tsp. of fine sea salt

1. Preheat oven to 325°F. Line a rimmed baking sheet with parchment paper.
2. Combine all the ingredients except the maple syrup in a large mixing bowl. Stir well and slowly pour in maple syrup as you continue to mix.
3. Spread onto parchment paper.
4. Bake for 10 minutes, then toss around and bake for another 10 minutes.
5. Allow to cool at room temperature before storing in airtight container (mason jars).

(Makes 4 servings.)

▶ **Lunch**

Brown Rice and Kale Bowl

Brown rice and kale make the perfect base for your most imaginative vegetable creations. Kale is packed with more nutritional benefits and fewer calories than most foods around. This green leafy vegetable is loaded with phytonutrients that protect against cancers, and is also rich in fiber, calcium, vitamins A, C, B_6, and E, and manganese and copper. Kale is truly a nutrient superstar!

INGREDIENTS:

1 cup of brown rice

kale

vegetables of choice

1. Rinse brown rice under water for 30 seconds.
2. Place rice in a pot with 2 cups of water. Bring to a boil, cover, and simmer for 40 minutes, or until the liquid has been absorbed and the rice is soft.
3. Place cooked rice in a bowl of kale and top with raw vegetables of choice (broccoli, cucumber, tomatoes, carrots, etc.).
4. Use lemon/lime juice as dressing, or mix 2 tbsp. of balsamic vinegar with 1 tbsp. of mustard and a dash of pepper for a homemade balsamic vinaigrette.

▶ Dinner

Tomato and Avocado Salad

Simple, gorgeous, packed with freshness and with health: an instant classic.

INGREDIENTS:

2 medium tomatoes

1 Haas avocado

2 limes, juiced

2 tsp. dried basil leaves

1 tbsp. extra virgin olive oil (optional)

sea salt, to taste

ground black pepper, to taste

1. Wash and dry tomatoes, then chop and set aside in a mixing bowl.
2. Cut avocado in half, peel the skin, slice in cubes, and combine with tomatoes.

Recipe Continues

3. Add the lime juice, basil, olive oil, sea salt, and pepper, and lightly toss together.

4. This salad can be enjoyed as a complete meal or as a snack, making this 2 servings.

EXERCISE

CARDIO: Do 30–45 minutes of the cardio of your choice (suggestions outlined on page 222), followed by 10–15 minutes of stretching.

DAY 10

GO FOR 100 PERCENT

By day ten, you should be experiencing some weight loss; the amount depends on your starting weight and overall fitness level. If you aren't losing weight, you need to take a closer look at what you are *really* putting into your mouth, not what you intended to put in your mouth. It's just too easy to graze all day and not realize it! And grazing and denial go hand in hand. Take an honest account of how well you're following the plan.

Most of the people I talk to who feel like they have an inability to lose weight honestly believe that they don't eat very much. In their heart, they truly believe they're not eating, because this mindless grazing is such a deeply ingrained habit. So I know I need to get specific and walk through a day with them: "What did you eat for breakfast? What did you eat for lunch? Did you have any snacks in between?" And then the truth slips out.

"Well, I guess I did have, like, a little wine. And then I had a couple of brownies yesterday. And yeah, my weakness is chocolate, so sometimes . . ."

And there you have it: the denial of the habit, denial of the automatic response—the same habit that is subverting all of their plans for success. That's why you have to go for 100 percent. When you go for 100 percent, denial doesn't even have room to slip in. Ninety-five percent makes room. Seventy-five percent makes room.

If you want to succeed, go for 100 percent!

DAY 10 MENU

▶ **Breakfast**

All You Need Is a Cape Juice

Ginger is an herb that has been used by people as a spice and a medicine since prehistoric times[55] *and was one of the most important spices in medieval times.*[56] *It is used to treat stomach issues like motion sickness and morning sickness, nausea, and vomiting; muscle soreness; arthritis; coughs; and bronchitis. It appears that the chemicals in ginger work by reducing inflammation and nausea in the stomach and intestines, but it is possible that they control feelings of nausea in the brain.*

> **MIX ALL INGREDIENTS IN A BLENDER UNTIL SMOOTH:**
>
> 1 handful of spinach
> 2 stalks of kale
> 1 cucumber
> 1 lemon
> ½ inch of gingerroot
> 1 inch of whole turmeric (or 1 tsp. of powdered if fresh is not available)
> 1 pinch parsley
> 2 carrots
> 1 Granny Smith apple (cored)

▶ **Lunch**

Raw Walnut Tacos

Creativity is encouraged so feel free to make this one your own using almonds or any combination of mixed nuts!

---

[55] Harold McGee, *On Food and Cooking*, 425.

[56] Ibid.

TACO MEAT INGREDIENTS:

2 cups nuts

2 heads of romaine lettuce

1½ tbsp. cumin

1 tbsp. coriander

2 tbsp. balsamic vinegar

1 tbsp. coconut aminos

dash paprika

dash garlic powder

dash black ground pepper

GARNISH INGREDIENTS:

2 Haas avocados

½ pint cherry tomatoes (1 small pack)

½ tbsp. dried parsley flakes

pinch black ground pepper

pinch sea salt

1 lime

1. Thoroughly wash and drain the lettuce and tomatoes in a colander or on a paper towel and set aside while preparing remaining ingredients.
2. Combine all taco ingredients in a food processor.
3. Pulse several times until crumbly, making sure not to overblend.
4. Spread the nut taco meat on the romaine leaves in 4 equal servings.
5. Slice tomatoes in halves.
6. Slice the avocados in half and remove the pit. Peel the skin and cut into small, even pieces.
7. Garnish the nut taco meat with sliced avocado, tomatoes, parsley, ground pepper, sea salt, and lime juice.

▶ **Dinner**

Black Bean and Kale Salad

Marilyn knows that whenever she makes this salad, I get a huge smile on my face. So she's nice enough to make it often! The fennel adds a crisp crunch with light licorice flavor. You don't have to know the words rutin, quercetin, and kaempferol glycosides to be assured that the fennel you sliced into your lunch is full of antioxidants that help your body fight free radicals (but now you do).[57]

INGREDIENTS:

1 cup black beans, uncooked (or 1 cup canned)
4 cups water
2 cups kale, finely chopped
¾ cup tomato, diced
¼ cup curly parsley, diced
½ Haas avocado, chopped
⅓ cup fennel, diced
¼ cup onion, diced
⅓ cup carrots, shredded
1 tbsp. extra virgin olive oil
3 tbsp. lemon juice
sea salt and pepper, to taste

DIRECTIONS FOR COOKING BLACK BEANS:

1. Presoak 1 cup black beans overnight in 4 cups of cold water to reduce cooking time, or quick-soak (cover beans with water, bring to a boil for 2 minutes, then remove from heat and let sit for 1–2 hours).

2. Rinse, drain, then cover with 3 cups of fresh water and continue cooking.

3. Bring water and beans to a boil, reduce heat, cover, and let simmer, skimming off any foam and stirring occasionally (presoaked beans will take about 1 hour to cook).

---

[57] http://www.whfoods.com/genpage.php?tname=foodspice&dbid=23, accessed July 24, 2014.

4. Beans are done when tender.

5. Rinse and drain. Unused beans can be stored in an airtight container or in heavy-duty freezer bags for 3–4 days, or in freezer for 1–2 months.

DIRECTIONS FOR SALAD:

1. In a mixing bowl, add 1 cup cooked black beans, kale, tomato, parsley, avocado, fennel, onion, carrots, olive oil, and lemon juice, and lightly mix together.

2. Add sea salt and pepper, to taste, and serve!

EXERCISE

■ **RESISTANCE TRAINING:** Complete the exercises outlined on page 222.

DAY 11

EARN YOUR REWARDS

■

As a society, we've become so comfortable that we've lost sight of what it is to truly work for something. Before credit cards existed, what did you have to do? You had to work really hard for something before you could get it. Now you don't. Now you can just use a card before you have earned something, and then you're paying it off for the next four years.

That's what we're doing with our food.

When you abuse a credit card, the reality is that you've just given yourself something that you haven't earned. That you haven't worked for yet. That behavior is so deeply ingrained that we treat our whole lives that way, financially and nutritionally: always rewarding ourselves, even though we haven't earned it. And then paying it off over years, with worry and poor health.

The goal of the 22-Day Revolution is to make you conscious and aware: conscious about food, aware of when you eat and what you are eating, so you can stop using food as a reward. So you can give yourself the real reward: good health and vitality.

If you find yourself feeling frustrated or wanting to "reward" yourself with food that isn't on the plan, hit pause. Did you earn this reward? Or are you borrowing energy you won't be able to pay back—which will lead to weight gain instead of loss, and poor health instead of good health?

For optimal health (and a better credit report), earn your rewards. Don't borrow them.

▶ **Breakfast**

French Toast

French toast in a diet book? That's right. With the right ingredients, you can enjoy your favorite foods and still give yourself the health benefits of eating plants!

INGREDIENTS:

    4 slices of vegan and gluten-free bread

    1 ripe banana

    1½ cups of almond milk

▲ ½ tbsp. milled flaxseed

    1 dash cinnamon

    ½ tsp. vanilla

1. In a large mixing bowl mash banana.

2. Add almond milk, vanilla, cinnamon, and flax and stir.

3. Coat skillet with coconut oil and preheat to medium.

4. Once your skillet is hot, dip your slices into the mixture and flip to ensure both sides are completely covered.

5. Cook until golden brown on each side.

6. Serve immediately and top with maple syrup.

▶ **Lunch**

Cauliflower Salad

INGREDIENTS:

    1 medium head cauliflower

    1 lemon (juice)

    dash salt

    dash pepper

Recipe Continues

2 tbsp. pine nuts

½ cup grapes (sliced in half)

1. Heat oven to 300 degrees.
2. In a mixing bowl toss the cauliflower with all the ingredients.
3. Place on parchment paper and roast for 15–30 minutes.

▶ **Dinner**

Kale Salad with Sweet Potato

Two of my favorites—united! The sharp bite of the kale with the sweetness of the sweet potato is an amazing combo, especially when you add cranberries and sunflower seeds . . . which also help to up the nutritional value. It doesn't get better than this!

INGREDIENTS:

1 small sweet potato

1 handful of kale

¼ cup dried cranberries

¼ cup sunflower seeds

dash sea salt

2 tbsp. balsamic vinegar

1 tbsp. mustard

1. Preheat the oven to 350 degrees.
2. Scrub sweet potato under running water and steam until tender.
3. Place sweet potato on parchment paper and bake for 10 minutes, or until edges are crisp.
4. Chop kale and toss with sweet potato, cranberries, and sunflower seeds.
5. Whisk mustard, vinegar, and salt together and drizzle over the top.

EXERCISE

■ **CARDIO:** Do 30–45 minutes of the cardio of your choice (suggestions outlined on page 222), followed by 10–15 minutes of stretching.

DAY 12

REMEMBER THAT YOU'RE IN THE DRIVER'S SEAT

Food and fitness are areas of our lives where we have the most autonomy, and we practice the least amount of it. Imagine a road blocked by a huge tree, and your brakes are working just fine. Yet, all around me, I see people driving toward that tree, and they just refuse to take their foot off the gas or turn the wheel.

Other people, your boss, the weather: You have no control over any of that. But you do have control over much more than you realize: your health, how you feel, how you look, how you age. Your energy levels. How you sleep. But instead of exercising control in these few areas that are within our grasp, we allow ourselves to be swayed by those fears that demand the immediate comfort food gives us. Don't you really want the long-term comfort of feeling healthy, fit, and happy? Of losing weight, reversing disease, clearing up your skin, protecting your vision, and so many other things?

We just have to stop being afraid of what will happen if we succeed: that we might have to change, that we might have to grow, that we might have to be uncomfortable on the way there. We have to cut through the psychological layers that are holding us back. Do you know what the difference between a winner and a loser is? Nothing. The loser just hasn't won yet. Anybody can be a winner. You have to keep trying. And when you make that first shot, even if you missed those first ten, as soon as you make that first basket—*whoom*, you get another one.

And you just became a winner.

You're in charge! Practice the discipline that you need to be able to live the best you.

DAY 12 MENU

▶ **Breakfast**

Extra C Juice

MIX ALL INGREDIENTS IN A BLENDER UNTIL SMOOTH:

1 orange

4 carrots

4 stalks of celery

1 lemon

½-inch (raw ginger)

▶ **Lunch**

Thin-Crust Pizza

Add extra veggies like onions and peppers for toppings with a punch.

INGREDIENTS FOR CRUST:

¾ cup brown-rice flour

½ cup tapioca flour

⅓ cup water

1 tsp. olive oil

½ tsp. sea salt

INGREDIENTS FOR TOPPINGS:

2 medium ripe tomatoes

½ Haas avocado

2 fresh basil leaves, chopped (or 1 tsp. dried basil flakes)

black ground pepper, to taste

Recipe Continues

INGREDIENTS FOR VEGAN MOZZARELLA CHEESE:

- ½ cup raw cashews, soaked
- 1 cup water
- 1 tbsp. tapioca flour
- 1 tsp. lemon juice
- 1 tsp. apple cider vinegar
- ½ tsp. sea salt, or to taste

1. To prepare the cheese, add all ingredients into a high-speed blender and blend until creamy. In a saucepan, cook the cheese, stirring often over medium-high heat. Reduce heat and keep stirring to prevent burning. Once consistency has thickened (looks like melted cheese), remove from heat and let cool. Set aside while preparing other ingredients. Leftovers can be stored in fridge up to 5–7 days.
2. Preheat oven to 350. Lightly grease and dust a baking sheet or pizza stone with brown-rice flour.
3. In a mixing bowl, combine the flours with the salt and whisk together.
4. Make a well in the center and add the water and oil and mix with a spoon. If necessary, add 1 tbsp. at a time of water until consistency is reached.
5. Scoop out the dough onto a baking sheet or pizza stone and use hands to shape and press down into desired shape (square/rectangular). Smooth with wet fingers and prebake for about 20–25 minutes.
6. Wash and slice each tomato into 3 thick slices.
7. Remove the pizza crust from the oven and top with the 6 slices of tomato, sliced avocado, cheese (or vegan cheese of choice), and basil.
8. Bake for another 15–20 minutes until slightly crisp.
9. Remove from oven, top with a dash of pepper, slice into 6 square slices, and serve (serves 2)!

Lentil Burger with Veggies

My wife makes these burgers often, especially in summertime, when everybody's firing up the grill! Enjoy your lentil burger topped with avocado, tomato, lettuce, onion, and tahini sauce (mix 1 tbsp. tahini with 3 tbsp. lemon juice and a dash of sea salt) on vegan and gluten-free bread. Delicious!

INGREDIENTS:

    2 cups black lentils, cooked

▲ 2 cups quinoa, cooked (⅓ cup dry quinoa plus ⅔ cup of water)

    1 cup carrots, chopped

    ⅓ cup onion, chopped

    1 tbsp. lemon juice

    1 tbsp. arrowroot flour

    2 tbsp. garbanzo flour

    ¼ tsp. cumin

    ¼ tsp. coriander

    1 tbsp. parsley flakes, dried or fresh

    dash garlic powder

    ½ tsp. sea salt, or to taste

DIRECTIONS FOR COOKING BLACK LENTILS:

1. Rinse thoroughly with cold water in a sieve until water runs clear.

2. In a pot, combine 1 cup of black lentils with 4 cups of water and bring to a boil. Add a pinch of sea salt, bring to a simmer, and cover. Let cook for about 20 minutes, stirring occasionally, making sure not to overcook.

3. Remove from heat, drain, rinse, and set aside.

DIRECTIONS FOR QUINOA:

1. Rinse thoroughly with cold water in a sieve.

Recipe Continues

2. In a pot, combine 1 cup of quinoa with 2 cups of water and bring to a boil. Add a pinch of sea salt, bring to a simmer, and cover. Let cook for about 20 minutes. Once cooled, leftovers can be stored in the fridge for up to a week.

DIRECTIONS FOR BURGERS:

1. Preheat oven to 400°F.
2. In a food processor add onion, carrots, about 1 cup of quinoa, 1 cup of lentils and lemon juice.
3. Pulse well until evenly chopped. Then add the arrowroot, garbanzo flour, cumin, coriander, parsley, garlic, and sea salt and pulse again.
4. Add mixture to remaining quinoa and lentils and blend together.
5. Portion the mix into six even patties with the palms of your hands. Or, divide 12 patties if you want to make sliders.
6. Bake at 400 degrees on greased parchment paper for approximately 45 minutes, turning patty once at about 20 minutes. Can also be made on the stove.
7. Leftovers can be stored in the fridge for a few days, or in the freezer in an airtight container for up to 6 months. (Makes about 6 burgers.)

EXERCISE

■ **RESISTANCE TRAINING:** Complete the exercises outlined on page 222.

DAY 13

LEARN HOW TO SAY NO

Recently, my wife and I went to our son's school for an event. There was plenty of healthy food, and then, for dessert, there were neon-frosted cupcakes covered in sprinkles. While we stood there, a teacher approached one of the children and said, "Daniel, you haven't touched your cupcake!"

And he said, "No, thank you."

She said, "Why don't you just taste it?"

The seven-year-old said, "I don't want any."

And she said, "How do you know you won't like it if you don't try it?"

If she had been encouraging him to taste the broccoli, or have a piece of celery, I would have understood. But why was she trying to encourage him to eat this Day-Glo cake? It was completely mind-blowing.

There will always be people who want to offer you another cupcake, another plate of pasta, another heaping portion of something you don't need. It may be your boss, or your mother-in-law. Sometimes they will be close friends, and sometimes they will be authority figures.

It's still okay to say no, thanks. In fact, it's imperative to gather the strength to say no.

DAY 13

▶ Breakfast

Overnight Oats

A clever, no-cook way to get your breakfast in on even the busiest mornings . . . just put it in the fridge the night before!

INGREDIENTS:

- ▲ ½ cup of gluten-free oats
- ½ cup of almond milk
- 1 dash cinnamon
- ▲ ½ tbsp. milled flaxseed
- ½ cup fresh fruit

1. Mix oats, cinnamon, and almond milk in a bowl and store in a covered mason-type jar in the refrigerator overnight.
2. In the morning top with milled flaxseed and fresh fruit.

22 ways! *Get creative and top with different combinations of fresh fruit, seeds, and nuts.*

▶ Lunch

Quinoa Tabbouleh

Tabbouleh is traditionally made with cracked wheat. Here we use quinoa, so we get better nutrition, with all the flavor of the original.

INGREDIENTS:

- ▲ 1 cup quinoa
- ½ lemon
- 1 garlic clove, minced
- 1 dash ground pepper
- 1 cucumber, chopped

1 box cherry tomatoes, ½ pint quartered

1 pinch parsley flakes

1 scallion, chopped

dash salt

1. Rinse one cup of quinoa in a fine sieve, drain, and transfer to a medium pot.
2. Add 2 cups of water and a pinch of salt. Bring to a boil and simmer until the water is absorbed and quinoa is fluffy (15–20 minutes).
3. Meanwhile, mix together all other ingredients in a bowl.
4. Let quinoa cool. Then add to the mixture, toss, and coat with lemon juice, salt, and pepper.

▶ Dinner

Vegetable Curry

INGREDIENTS:

4 cups mixed veggies (any combination, or try broccoli, kale, peppers, cauliflower and spinach in equal servings)

1 onion, finely chopped

2 garlic cloves, chopped

1 tbsp. fresh ginger, grated

2 tsp. curry

dash salt

1 can coconut milk

1. In a large skillet over medium heat, sauté onions, garlic, and ginger in a dime-size dollop of canola oil for 2 minutes.
2. Add in all the other ingredients and bring to a simmer until the sauce thickens and the veggies are tender.

EXERCISE:

■ **CARDIO:** Do 30–45 minutes of the cardio of your choice (suggestions outlined on page 222), followed by 10–15 minutes of stretching.

KEEP PEDALING

■

Today marks the end of two weeks, and the beginning of week three, your final stretch. You should be feeling elated by now—you've been working so hard, and you're already experiencing the benefits of eating plants: You've lost weight, you have more energy, people around you keep commenting on your glow.

But that doesn't mean it's easy. Elation sometimes comes from knowing you are fighting the good fight. Temptation will always be there. And so will your commitment to working through it.

I have a really cool friend who is like a mentor to me, and I always take his wisdom to heart. He says that life is like riding a bicycle: If you're not pedaling, you fall. If you're moving really quickly and you aren't pedaling, you're probably going in the wrong direction—downhill. When you're pedaling and it's hard, that's how you know you're making progress.

So keep pedaling!

DAY 14 MENU

▶ **Breakfast**

Clarity Juice

Beets lend a gorgeous hue and sweet taste to juices. They're also superpowered for your health. According to some studies, drinking beet juice can help boost stamina so you can exercise longer. It can also help to lower blood pressure.[58]

MIX ALL INGREDIENTS IN A BLENDER UNTIL SMOOTH:

1 cucumber

1 apple

1 lemon (peeled)

1 pinch parsley

2 beets

▶ **Lunch**

Vegan Sushi Roll

INGREDIENTS:

1 cup short-grain brown rice, cooked

½ Haas avocado, cut in two slices

3 tbsp. jicama, ground in food processor

2 tbsp. raw spinach, ground in food processor

2 tbsp. raw carrots, ground in food processor

▲ 2 tbsp. crushed cashews

1 tbsp. light canola mayo

sesame seeds

1 nori sheet

sushi bamboo mat

Recipe Continues

---

[58] http://www.webmd.com/food-recipes/features/truth-about-beetroot-juice, accessed July 22, 2014.

1. Cover the bamboo mat with plastic wrap.
2. Place the nori with the rough side facing upward.
3. Wet hands and place the brown rice in the middle of the nori. Evenly spread the rice with fingers while pressing down gently.
4. Flip the nori over and place the avocado slices across the middle of the nori, along with the broccoli, cauliflower, mayo, and cashews.
5. Begin to roll the mat, keeping it tight with every move forward, including the sides.
6. Sprinkle sesame seeds and, with a wet knife, cut the roll into 6–8 pieces and enjoy!

▶ **Dinner**

Quinoa-Stuffed Red Peppers

There's just something gorgeous about stuffed peppers—it's the kind of dish that gets "oohs" when you bring it to the table. This version gets "oohs" after everybody takes a bite, too. And they're so good for you! A cup of peppers gives you all you need of vitamins A and C for the day. The more colors of peppers you enjoy, the more varied the phytochemicals you get. Red bell peppers are rich in phytochemicals like lutein and zeaxanthin, which may be useful for eye diseases; beta-carotene, which may help fight some types of cancer; and lycopene, which some think can decrease the risk for ovarian cancer.[59]

INGREDIENTS:

▲ 1 cup quinoa
1 BPA-free can of pinto beans
4 medium peppers
1 small sweet onion
½ tbsp. cumin
dash salt
dash garlic powder
dash pepper

[59] http://www.webmd.com/food-recipes/features/health-benefits-of-peppers, accessed July 24, 2014.

1. Preheat oven to 350 degrees.
2. Cut peppers open through the top and remove seeds.
3. Rinse one cup of quinoa in a fine sieve, drain, and transfer to a medium pot.
4. Add 2 cups of water and a pinch of salt. Bring to a boil and simmer until the water is absorbed and quinoa is fluffy (15–20 minutes).
5. Toss beans, onion, garlic, cumin, salt, and pepper in a bowl and mix with quinoa.
6. Stuff peppers with quinoa/bean mix, place on a baking sheet covered with parchment paper, and bake for 20–25 minutes.

(Serving: Make one to two peppers per person depending on size. If they're about the size of your fist, two; if they're much bigger, one)

EXERCISE

■ **RESISTANCE TRAINING:** Complete the exercises outlined on page 222.

11

WEEK 3:
DEVELOPING AWARENESS

WELCOME TO WEEK THREE! YOU'VE already done a lot of hard work to incorporate fresh foods into your diet, to change those ingrained habits, and to be consistent and show up every day. By now it should be feeling a little more natural to wake up to mouthwatering raspberries and blueberries and lunch on those gorgeous green salads. So I think you're ready for something a little bit more subtle: awareness.

You will have opportunities to be aware of your food before, during, and after your meals.

- *Be conscious of your food before you eat.* What are you going to eat at your next meal? Do you have fresh foods available? Have you done the necessary planning?
- *Be conscious of your food while you eat.* Are you sitting in a place where you feel relaxed, with some time to focus on your meal? How does the food taste? Is it crispy, chewy, sour, sweet? Have you had the right amount to eat? Are you satisfied, but not too full?
- *Be conscious of your food after you eat.* The real reward of food is how good it can make you feel!

Being conscious and being obsessive are not the same things! People on diets sometimes feel that the best way to succeed is by creating a rigid formula for success, like counting calories. By obsessing on these numbers, it can feel like you are taking control of your destiny. But for how long does a program like that really last? Unless you are a mathematician, endlessly counting and adding and multiplying isn't very much fun, and can distract you from being really present at meals.

Instead of counting calories, I'd like you to focus on *kaizen*. *Kaizen*, which means "change for the best," is a Japanese concept for small improvements. The idea of *kaizen* has found itself a home in big business. In manufacturing and engineering, *kaizen* is used to identify the places where mistakes are made or where systems could run more smoothly. It encourages us to look more closely and adopt tiny, effective shifts that can have a huge ripple effect.

This kind of thinking is as useful small-scale as it is large-scale. In a city, *kaizen* thinking and observing can be the difference between a block covered with litter because there is no trash can, and visible trash cans that encourage people to put their refuse where it belongs. At home, *kaizen* can mean making fruit and vegetables as convenient as packaged goods by rinsing and slicing produce before you store it for easy access and easy eating. It can mean taking a different route home so that you no longer pass by your favorite bakery every single day. It can mean learning to push back from the table before you feel stuffed, rather than lingering and finishing every bite on your plate and the plates around you.

Instead of obsessing, *kaizen* encourages us to reflect and consider. What are the triggers that influence your daily habits? What are the habits that are helping you succeed—or derailing you? This week, how can you focus on using awareness to tweak your patterns to lead you toward achievement, empowerment, and health?

RECOGNIZE FULLNESS

With all the advancements in technology, life has gotten really, really fast. Too many of us have gotten into the habit of eating too quickly, eating at our desks, or not having lunch whatsoever. And when we eat, we eat so fast that we don't allow our bodies to tell us when we've gotten to that point where we are full. It's like when you're filling your car with gas. You stop when you're almost there; you don't allow the gas to overflow.

If you are overweight, more than likely it's because when you eat, you overfill the tank and allow the gas to come over the top. How many times have you walked away from a meal thinking, *I probably should have stopped a few bites ago.*

Focus on how you *really* feel after meals. Because if you pushed away from every meal feeling, *You know, I could take a few more bites but I'm good. I'm in that place where I feel really good*, you'd be a healthy weight.

Over time, I've found that the absolute healthiest way to eat is to 80 percent fullness, or just a little bit less than full. Twenty minutes after a meal, when your body has had a chance to begin digesting and processing your hunger level, you're perfect. Our bodies are very sophisticated, amazing machines, but in this technological world of immediate, at-your-fingertips gratification, we need to be patient. If you're not patient, and you take those extra three bites so you can feel satisfied immediately, you'll regret it. You won't feel well, your stomach will hurt, and you'll feel lethargic—all of which are the opposite of your intentions when you sit down for a meal.

Really, your food should make you feel like you're ready to go! Remember to practice restraint if you really want to enjoy your food.

DAY 15 MENU

▶ **Breakfast**

On-the-Run Protein Smoothie

On the run? No problem. Pour into a travel cup and take with you for a protein-packed punch that will keep you running for as long as you need.

2 scoops 22 Days plant-based protein powder (chocolate)

2 cups almond milk

1 frozen banana

1 tbsp. sunflower butter

▶ **Lunch**

Black Bean and Kale Salad

INGREDIENTS:

1 cup black beans, uncooked (or 1 cup canned)

3 cups water

2 cups kale, finely chopped

¾ cup tomato, diced

¼ cup curly parsley, diced

½ Haas avocado, chopped

⅓ cup fennel, diced

¼ cup onion, diced

⅓ cup carrots, shredded

1 tbsp. extra virgin olive oil

3 tbsp. lemon juice

sea salt and pepper, to taste

DIRECTIONS FOR COOKING BLACK BEANS:

1. Presoak 1 cup black beans overnight in 4 cups of cold water to reduce cooking time, or quick-soak (cover beans with water, bring to a boil for 2 minutes, then remove from heat and let sit for 1–2 hours).
2. Rinse, drain, then cover with 3 cups of fresh water and continue cooking.
3. Bring water and beans to a boil, reduce heat, cover, and let simmer, skimming off any foam and stirring occasionally (presoaked beans will take about 1 hour to cook).
4. Beans are done when tender.
5. Rinse and drain. Unused beans can be stored in an airtight container or in heavy-duty freezer bags for 3–4 days, or in freezer for 1–2 months.

DIRECTIONS FOR SALAD:

1. In a mixing bowl, add 1 cup cooked black beans, kale, tomato, parsley, avocado, fennel, onion, carrots, olive oil, and lemon juice, and lightly mix together.
2. Add sea salt and pepper, to taste, and serve!

▶ **Dinner**

Ceviche

You'll love this recipe for a quiet dinner, or for a dinner party. Your guests will go crazy for it! Carrots lend a burst of orange as well as 203 percent of your daily supply of vitamin A in just one serving, and plenty of potassium. And spicy peppers, like the jalapeño, are full of a chemical called capsaicin, found in the white pith on the inside of the pepper. Capsaicin raises the body's temperature, makes you sweat, and increases your metabolic rate. It can also make you feel less hungry.[60]

Recipe Continues

---

[60] Harold McGee *On Food and Cooking*, 419.

INGREDIENTS:

2 cups hearts of palm, sliced

1 Haas avocado, diced

1 cup cucumber, diced

1 cup carrots, diced

½ cup scallions, diced

1 small jalapeño, seeded and minced

4 limes, juiced

1 tbsp. extra virgin olive oil, optional

dash parsley flakes

dash sea salt

dash ground black pepper

1. In a mixing bowl, combine the hearts of palm, avocado, cucumber, carrots, scallions, jalapeño, lime juice, and olive oil.
2. Gently mix together and serve.
3. Top with parsley flakes, sea salt, and pepper. (Serves 2.)

EXERCISE

■ **CARDIO:** Do 30–45 minutes of the cardio of your choice (suggestions outlined on page 222), followed by 10–15 minutes of stretching.

DAY 16

KEEP AN EYE ON YOURSELF

Medicine is the science of observation. Doctors observe. But who better to observe us than us? You know what makes you feel good. You know what makes you eat. You know that if you get stressed out, you reach for that chocolate bar. You know that when you deserve a reward you head straight for the ice cream. And if you don't know these things about yourself, stop and take the time to catalog the cravings and the patterns. Be honest with yourself. This is the time to acknowledge the old habits that have been holding you back, and work toward creating new, healthier habits.

Now, use your awareness to create those new habits. You have to figure out just what triggers those automatic responses in order to find the alternative response that falls in line with what you're going toward. You have to figure out better ways to reward yourself. You have to turn automatic responses into conscious choices!

Let's say that at three thirty every day, you suddenly get the funny feeling that you need to get up from your desk and have a snack. So you do—you need a break and so you get up and wander around the room for a moment and get a brownie from the vending machine or the café down the block. Of course, ten minutes later you are regretting that brownie, and then you feel guilty instead of great. Why did you get up from your desk originally? Because you felt a little antsy, and all you wanted was to feel better. Instead, you feel worse.

This is a great moment for change. Peel back the intentions behind rising from your desk. Was it hunger? Nope. Was it boredom? Maybe. Or maybe you just needed to get up and move around. Once you've uncovered the real reason for your daily brownie—a break!—you can plan a better way. You can plan to get up at three thirty and step outside, not to buy a brownie, but just to breathe in some fresh air, because all you really needed was a little space from work to give your brain a moment to clear. *It was never about the brownie!* It was about taking five minutes to get reinspired, refocused, realigned so you could get back to work—with no regrets, just the amazing feeling that you take great care of yourself whether you're at work or at home.

Observe yourself so that you can catch yourself in the act—and then shift that action to something that will give you what you're really looking for.

DAY 16 MENU

▶ Breakfast

Alive Juice

Fresh turmeric is a relative of ginger. It looks like its cousin but comes in a vibrant yellow hue. You'll find it fresh in our recipes for our juices because it has so many benefits . . . among them helping to alleviate arthritis, stomach pain, bloating, colds, and headaches. It is thought that the chemicals in turmeric might decrease swelling and inflammation.[61]

MIX ALL INGREDIENTS IN A BLENDER UNTIL SMOOTH:

- 4 stalks of kale
- 1 cucumber
- 1 cup pineapple
- 2 stalks celery
- 1 inch turmeric

▶ Lunch

Hummus Tartine with Sprouts

A tartine is an open-faced sandwich, and this fabulous rendition begins with hummus and then piles on the veggies for a beautiful treat. It takes only two minutes to make, and it's easy to bring with you on the run and to work.

Recipe Continues

---

[61] http://www.webmd.com/vitamins-supplements/ingredientmono-662-TURMERIC. aspx?activeIngredientId=662&activeIngredientName=TURMERIC&source=2, accessed July 22, 2014.

INGREDIENTS:

2 slices vegan and gluten-free bread

½ small Haas avocado

2 tbsp. hummus

1 pinch of alfalfa sprouts

4 cherry tomatoes

dash paprika

1. Spread hummus on toasted bread.
2. Top with sprouts, sliced tomatoes, and avocado and finish with a dash of paprika.

▶ **Dinner**

Lentil Soup Garnished with Avocado and Tomato

SOUP INGREDIENTS:

1½ cups dry green lentils

6 cups water

1 tbsp. high-heat safflower oil (or canola oil)

½ onion, finely chopped

¼ tsp. garlic, minced

½ tbsp. cumin

½ tsp. coriander

¼ tsp. turmeric

½ tsp. sea salt

dash cayenne pepper

GARNISH INGREDIENTS:

2 Haas avocados, chopped

3 plum tomatoes, diced

½ lemon, juiced

½ tsp. parsley, minced

dash sea salt

1. In a bowl, mix together all the garnish ingredients and set aside while preparing the lentil soup.
2. Sift through lentils, and rinse well in a colander, making sure to remove any tiny stones that may be mixed in.
3. In a saucepan, heat the safflower oil over medium heat. Add onion, garlic, and a dash of salt, making sure to stir occasionally until onion becomes translucent.
4. Add remaining soup ingredients and bring to a boil.
5. Reduce to a simmer, cover, and cook for about 45 minutes.
6. Stir occasionally to avoid the soup burning or sticking to the pot.
7. Once lentils are soft and tender and desired consistency is reached, serve and garnish.

(about 4 servings)

EXERCISE:

■ **RESISTANCE TRAINING:** Complete the exercises outlined on page 222.

DAY 17

ONE COUNTS

■

Let's face it: When you're dieting, no one action is going to lead to morbid obesity. No one action, no one snack, no one doughnut. You don't gain 100 pounds by eating one piece of cake or one doughnut! But if your habit is to join your colleagues every afternoon at the doughnut shop, what is that "one" doughnut doing to your diet, to your weight, to your health, to your resolve?

It's the perpetuation of the action, not the first bite. You don't stay overweight from one cookie. You don't get Type 2 diabetes from one ice-cream sundae. You don't have a heart attack from one cheeseburger.

But if you never say no to the first bite, if you keep perpetuating the action, you're never going to lose weight, and you're probably going to gain it.

Unfortunately, the truth is that one choice leads to the next. Good choices lead to more good choices. Poor choices lead to more poor choices. You eat a bag of potato chips at night and you wake up feeling puffy and like crap. So you might as well have a doughnut instead of a green smoothie, right?

It isn't until you take yourself off the hamster wheel that you can free yourself. Each choice matters, because each choice leads to the next choice. If you want to start that thousand-mile journey, you can't weep over how long it will be: you have to start! You have to take that first step! Every choice is a step toward your future. What kind of future do you want to secure for yourself?

So pick up that foot. Walk to the salad bar. Take a different route home from dinner so you don't pass that bakery if you can't drive by without pulling into the parking lot. Keep the cookies out of the pantry if you can't resist eating them once you get home.

Your journey started with one step, and each subsequent step moves you either forward or backward.

Keep moving that foot forward!

DAY 17 MENU

▶ **Breakfast**

Tomato, Avocado, and Hummus Tartine

This one is topped with fruit for a delicious breakfast. Yes, you read that right. Like tomatoes, avocados are often treated like a veggie, but they're really a fruit. Either way, avocados provide nearly 20 essential nutrients for your diet, like potassium, vitamin E, B vitamins, and folic acid. They can also help to boost the quality of the nutrition that you're eating alongside them by helping you absorb more fat-soluble nutrients, like alpha- and beta-carotene and lutein.[62]

INGREDIENTS:

> 2 slices of vegan and gluten-free bread
> ½ small Hass avocado
> 2 tbsp. hummus
> 4 cherry tomatoes
> 1 sprinkle of paprika

1. Spread hummus on toasted bread.
2. Top with sliced tomatoes and avocado and finish with a sprinkle of paprika.

▶ **Lunch**

Bean Medley over Sweet Potato

Another rich and satisfying sweet potato creation! Sweet potatoes are a great base for almost every topping. Choose any combination of nutrient-rich beans you have on hand, or try my favorite combination: navy beans and kidney beans.

---

[62] http://www.californiaavocado.com/nutrition/, accessed July 22, 2014.

INGREDIENTS:

- 1 sweet potato
- 1 cup bean medley (½ cup navy beans and ½ cup kidney beans, or any variety or combination)
- ½ small onion chopped
- 1 glove garlic chopped
- 1 dash salt
- ½ tsp. oregano
- 1 tsp. cumin
- 1½ tbsp. balsamic vinegar
- dash black ground pepper

1. Soak beans overnight. Drain, rinse, and discard water.

2. Place the beans in a medium pot with 4 cups of water, onion, garlic, oregano, and cumin and bring to a boil, then simmer for 45 minutes.

3. Once beans are tender, add vinegar, salt, and ground pepper.

4. Preheat oven to 450 degrees.

5. Scrub sweet potato under running water and dry.

6. Poke a few holes around the potato and place on a sheet of parchment paper.

7. Place sweet potato in the oven for 30 minutes and flip over for another 20 minutes.

8. Remove cooked potato from oven and slice in half after it has cooled a bit.

9. Top with black beans and garnish with tomato and avocado.

▶ **Dinner**

Artichoke, Tomato, and Avocado Salad

INGREDIENTS:

- 1 box grape tomatoes
- 1 Haas avocado
- 1 BPA-free can artichoke hearts
- 1 lemon
- 2 tbsp. Kalamata olives
- dash paprika

Recipe Continues

1. Into a mixing bowl, slice grape tomatoes into fourths, slice artichoke, peel avocado and chop into equal-size pieces.
2. Add in olives and lemon juice and toss gently.
3. Place into serving bowl and top with paprika.

EXERCISE

■ **CARDIO:** Do 30–45 minutes of the cardio of your choice (suggestions outlined on page 222), followed by 10–15 minutes of stretching.

DAY 18

DENY DENIAL

Whenever I talk with people who are overweight, I hear it.

"I don't know why I'm not losing weight. I barely eat anything."

"Why aren't I seeing benefits? I'm mostly vegan."

"I had a salad at lunch and a stir-fry for dinner. I didn't even have breakfast!"

"It's my thyroid."

"It's my hormones."

What they are really saying is, "I'm in denial."

I have a friend who is always complaining about his digestive issues. His stomach hurts, and he's always uncomfortable, especially after meals. And I say, always, "You should go plant-based." It's something I encourage, especially for people I love. I don't want my friend to suffer; I want him to be his best.

When I dig deeper and ask about his "almost vegan" meals, the truth comes out.

"Do you have cheese?"

"Oh, yeah, I love cheese."

"'Cause that's one of the biggest disrupters of your digestive system."

"Ooh, I have a weakness for cheese. Yeah, I eat a lot of cheese."

"Would you say you eat cheese every day?"

"Oh, yeah, easily every day. Probably a couple times a day."

"You're not almost vegan."

Recognizing that you are in denial is a crucial step! You have to recognize that your habits may not be exactly what you think they are if you aren't getting the results you want. Then you have to become aware of what you're putting in your body, and put the right foods on your plate in the right amounts.

Deny the denial! Be aware!

▶ **Breakfast**

Breathe Juice

Recently researchers have begun to pay attention to cucumbers, because they contain certain lignans that are connected with a reduced risk of cardiovascular disease as well as reduced risk of breast cancer, uterine cancer, ovarian cancer, and prostate cancer. Fresh cucumber can help your body fight free radicals and inflammation, and it's likely also beneficial for your antioxidants. And these low-calorie vegetables are a great source of vitamin C, beta-carotene, and manganese.[63]

    4 stalks celery
    1 large cucumber
    2 lemons (peeled)
    1 handful spinach

▶ **Lunch**

Chickpea Sandwich

INGREDIENTS:

    2 slices of vegan, gluten-free bread
    1 BPA-free can of chickpeas
    ¼ cup celery (chopped)
    ¼ cup carrots (shredded)
    2 tbsp. canola mayo
    1 tbsp. whole-grain mustard
    1 romaine lettuce (head)
    1 small tomato
    pinch ground pepper

Recipe Continues

---

[63] http://www.whfoods.com/genpage.php?tname=foodspice&dbid=42, accessed July 22, 2014.

1. Place chickpeas, mayo and mustard in a food processor. Pulse a few times until blended well, but not too smooth.
2. Transfer to a bowl, and mix with the celery and carrots.
3. Place lettuce over toasted bread and top with chickpea spread.
4. Add tomato and a dash of pepper to finish.

▶ **Dinner**

Quinoa Tabbouleh

Tabbouleh is traditionally made with cracked wheat. Here we use quinoa, so we get better nutrition, with all the flavor of the original.

INGREDIENTS:

- 1 cup quinoa
- ½ lemon
- 1 garlic clove, minced
- 1 dash ground pepper
- 1 cucumber, chopped
- 1 box cherry tomatoes, ½ pint quartered
- 1 pinch parsley flakes
- 1 scallion, chopped
- dash salt

1. Rinse one cup of quinoa in a fine sieve, drain, and transfer to a medium pot.
2. Add 2 cups of water and a pinch of salt. Bring to a boil and simmer until the water is absorbed and quinoa is fluffy (15–20 minutes).
3. Meanwhile, mix together all other ingredients in a bowl.
4. Let quinoa cool. Then add to the mixture, toss, and coat with lemon juice, salt, and pepper.

EXERCISE

■ **RESISTANCE TRAINING:** Complete the exercises outlined on page 222.

DAY 19

EMPOWER YOURSELF AND OTHERS

All the work you've done over the past 18 days, all the willpower you're going to call upon this week, is going to have some amazing results—for you and for the people around you.

Imagine being at dinner with friends and the waiter comes over and says, "Can I offer you some dessert?" And then you look at your friend and you say, "What do you think?" And your friend says, "Nah, I'm good." And you say, "Right, I'm good too." It's easy. Your friend just made it easy for you to pass on dessert.

But if your friend had said, "I want a double fudge cake," you would likely agree to share it.

Because we all affect one another! Research has shown that people with heavy friends tend to be heavier. By getting more fit, you will show your friends that it is possible. You will set a positive example by taking the steps to improve your own health. By empowering yourself, you will empower others.

When you start making positive changes, as your friends see the benefits, as they observe the new light in your eye and the spring in your step, they are going to jump on board. They are going to say, "Tell me how!"

Because we all affect one another. Watch! While many dieters wish they had more community support, if you can keep making the inspiring choice, even if your friends and family don't get on board on day one, a few weeks later, they'll all be saying, "Wait, you're really doing this? I want to do this with you."

As you shift your own habits, your conscious actions are having profound effects on you, and they will have profound effects on your friends and the people you love the most.

DAY 19 MENU

▶ Breakfast

Orange You Happy Juice

Oranges have a health profile that includes nearly a day's worth of vitamin C in just one serving, with benefits for colds and cardiovascular disease, and a potential to lower cholesterol, protect respiratory health, and protect against rheumatoid arthritis.[64]

1 peeled grapefruit
2 peeled oranges
1 lemon
½ inch of ginger

▶ Lunch

Brown Rice and Kale Bowl

INGREDIENTS:

1 cup of brown rice
kale
vegetables of choice

1. Rinse brown rice under water for 30 seconds.
2. Place rice in a pot with 2 cups of water. Bring to a boil, cover, and simmer for 40 minutes, or until the liquid has been absorbed and the rice is soft.
3. Place cooked rice in a bowl of kale and top with raw vegetables of choice (broccoli, cucumber, tomatoes, carrots, etc.).
4. Use lemon/lime juice as dressing, or mix 2 tbsp. of balsamic vinegar with 1 tbsp. of mustard and a dash of pepper for a homemade balsamic vinaigrette.

---

[64] http://www.whfoods.com/genpage.php?tname=foodspice&dbid=37, accessed July 23, 2014.

▶ **Dinner**

Vegetable Curry

INGREDIENTS:

4 cups mixed veggies (any combination, or try broccoli, kale, peppers, cauliflower and spinach in equal servings)

1 onion, finely chopped

2 garlic cloves, chopped

1 tbsp. fresh ginger, grated

2 tsp. curry

dash salt

1 can coconut milk

1. In a large skillet over medium heat, sauté onions, garlic, and ginger in a dime-size dollop of canola oil for 2 minutes.
2. Add in all the other ingredients and bring to a simmer until the sauce thickens and the veggies are tender.

EXERCISE

■ **CARDIO:** Do 30–45 minutes of the cardio of your choice (suggestions outlined on page 222), followed by 10–15 minutes of stretching.

DAY 20

GOOD ENERGY IN, GOOD ENERGY OUT

By now you should be feeling the shifts that come from eating fruits and vegetables and grains—all of the life-giving foods that the earth gives to us. When plants grow, the sun shines, energy is absorbed from the air and through the soil, and nature's chemistry turns light into the food that gives you energy— pure, natural, healing energy that will change the way you live in the world.

When you eat meat, you are consuming energy that was probably raised and killed in a less than humane way. Footage of factory-raised animals is depressing and upsetting—how can you feel your best when your energy is coming from such an awful place?

Eating plants is better for the world you live in, too. Climate change has been linked to eating meat by many leading environmental organizations. According to the Environmental Defense Fund, if every American skipped one meal of chicken per week and substituted vegetarian foods instead, the carbon dioxide savings would equal that of taking 500,000 cars off U.S. roads. A little change goes a very long way, in your body and in the big wide world. Now, that's good car-ma!

On so many levels, choosing wellness and the conscious habit of eating plants instead of unconsciously filling your home and plate with processed foods that lead to disease is the reset that will affect *everything*. The ripple effect of powering your body with the right energy, in the form of plants, is wholly incredible.

DAY 20 MENU

▶ **Breakfast**

Lean Green Juice

MIX ALL INGREDIENTS IN A BLENDER UNTIL SMOOTH:

4 stalks of kale

1 handful of spinach

1 frozen banana

2 green apples

1 lemon (juiced)

▶ **Lunch**

Quinoa Salad with Lentils

INGREDIENTS:

▲ 1 cup quinoa

1 cup lentils

½ tsp. fine sea salt

1 tbsp. cumin

1 tbsp. coriander

1 large carrot

dash black ground pepper

handful of spinach

1. Rinse one cup of quinoa in a fine sieve, drain, and transfer to a medium pot.
2. Add 2 cups of water and a pinch of salt. Bring to a boil and simmer until the water is absorbed and quinoa is fluffy (15–20 minutes).
3. Rinse one cup of lentils and transfer into a medium pot.
4. Add 2 cups of water, 1 tbsp. of cumin, 1 tbsp. coriander, 1 large carrot (chopped), 1 dash of black ground pepper.
5. Bring to a boil and simmer for 20–30 minutes. Add water as needed to make sure the lentils are just barely covered.
6. Serve quinoa over a bed of spinach and top with lentils.

Baked Eggplant with Pico de Gallo

INGREDIENTS FOR EGGPLANT:

> 1 large eggplant
>
> 4 tbsp. olive oil (for coating eggplant)
>
> sea salt, to taste

INGREDIENTS FOR PICO DE GALLO:

> 1 Haas avocado, quartered, pitted, peeled, and chopped
>
> 2 medium tomatoes, diced
>
> 1 small onion, minced
>
> ½ jalapeño pepper, seeded and minced
>
> 2 limes, juiced
>
> 1 garlic clove, minced
>
> ¼ cup parsley, minced (can use cilantro instead)
>
> black ground pepper, to taste
>
> sea salt, to taste

1. Preheat oven to 450.
2. Wash and peel skin of eggplant, then slice into half-inch round slices.
3. Lightly brush each slice with olive oil on both sides and sprinkle with sea salt.
4. Place on a lined baking sheet in the oven for about 8–10 minutes on each side.
5. Prepare the pico de gallo by adding all the ingredients in a mixing bowl and lightly tossing together.
6. Once eggplant is cooked, serve and top each slice with pico de gallo and enjoy!

EXERCISE

■ **RESISTANCE TRAINING:** Complete the exercises outlined on page 222.

DAY 21

REAP THE BENEFITS

You've been eating plants for three weeks, which means you're giving yourself everything you need to look and feel your best! When you wake up in the morning, you have a little more energy. Your lunch doesn't put you to sleep anymore. The clothes you thought you would never wear are starting to fit again. You may even have become the person who tells other people about the values of a plant-based lifestyle . . . and guess what? They're listening! Why? Because they see the changes in you. The way you glow. The way your eyes shine. The way you have a little more enthusiasm, a little more confidence, a little more energy.

Because the way we live gets written all over our faces. Before, in your old life, when you ate processed, salty snacks without noticing, and takeout loaded with MSG, you were probably used to waking up with puffy eyes from all the sodium. Well, these days instead of consuming the ingredients for sad-looking skin, you've been giving yourself all the balanced nutrition you need to look bright-eyed and feel ready to go.

Your skin should be showing the glow, because cutting back on animal products also means skipping much of their saturated fats, which are notorious for clogging pores. Plus, many of the vitamins and minerals in fruits and veggies contribute to healthy skin. The lycopene in tomatoes, for example, helps protect your skin from sun damage, and the vitamin C in sweet potatoes smooths wrinkles by stimulating the production of collagen.

If you're loving the skin you're in, from your new, slimmer self to the glow on your face, keep eating plants and taking the best possible care of yourself, inside and out.

DAY 21 MENU

▶ **Breakfast**

Avocado Bruschetta

That's right—bruschetta for breakfast!

INGREDIENTS:

1 medium tomato, finely chopped

⅓ Haas avocado, finely chopped

⅓ small onion, diced

1 garlic clove, minced

2 tbsp. lemon juice

2 tsp. extra virgin olive oil

1 tsp. balsamic vinegar

1 fresh basil leaf, chopped (or pinch of dried basil)

sea salt, to taste

ground black pepper, to taste

2 vegan and gluten-free slices of toast (recipe above)

1. In a mixing bowl, toss together the tomato, avocado, onion, garlic, lemon juice, oil, vinegar, basil, salt, and pepper.
2. Toast the bread, top with tomatoes, and serve! (Serves 1–2.)

▶ **Lunch**

Raw Walnut Tacos

Another opportunity to make this one your own using any combination of mixed nuts!

Recipe Continues

TACO MEAT INGREDIENTS:

2 cups nuts

2 heads of romaine lettuce

1½ tbsp. cumin

1 tbsp. coriander

2 tbsp. balsamic vinegar

1 tbsp. coconut aminos

dash paprika

dash garlic powder

dash black ground pepper

GARNISH INGREDIENTS:

2 Haas avocados

½ pint cherry tomatoes (1 small pack)

½ tbsp. dried parsley flakes

pinch black ground pepper

pinch sea salt

1 lime

1. Thoroughly wash and drain the lettuce and tomatoes in a colander or on a paper towel and set aside while preparing remaining ingredients.
2. Combine all taco ingredients in a food processor.
3. Pulse several times until crumbly, making sure not to overblend.
4. Spread the nut taco meat on the romaine leaves in 4 equal servings.
5. Slice tomatoes in halves.
6. Slice the avocados in half and remove the pit. Peel the skin and cut into small, even pieces.
7. Garnish the nut taco meat with sliced avocado, tomatoes, parsley, ground pepper, sea salt, and lime juice.

▶ **Dinner**

Kale Salad with Sweet Potato

Make this dish sing with creative toppings like cranberries and pumpkin or sunflower seeds.

INGREDIENTS:

> 1 small sweet potato
>
> 1 handful of kale
>
> ¼ cup dried cranberries
>
> ¼ cup sunflower seeds or pumpkin
>
> dash sea salt
>
> 2 tbsp. balsamic vinegar
>
> 1 tbsp. mustard

1. Preheat the oven to 350 degrees.
2. Scrub sweet potato under running water and steam until tender.
3. Place sweet potato on parchment paper and bake for 10 minutes, or until edges are crisp.
4. Chop kale and toss with sweet potato and your combination of cranberries and seeds.
5. Whisk mustard, vinegar, and salt together and drizzle over the top.

EXERCISE

■ **CARDIO:** Do 30–45 minutes of the cardio of your choice (suggestions outlined on page 222), followed by 10–15 minutes of stretching.

12

DAY 22:
THE BEGINNING OF THE BEST OF YOUR LIFE

HOW DID YOU FEEL WHEN you woke up this morning? I asked you that back on day one, and I'm asking again, because this is another kind of day one—day one of the best of your life.

How much better do you feel in your body than you did before you started the program? How much stronger? More vital? More alive?

You've shown up every day and given this your all. You've taken the steps you needed to really see your habits, deny your denial, and create newer, stronger, life- and health-giving habits.

Congratulations! I'm so proud of you, and I hope that you're proud of yourself. Today I'd like you to think about how you might make some of these habits into permanent, lasting ones. And it's not about living on a "diet." Maintaining a healthy weight is about shifting the way you think about the food you eat. Forget deprivation! Give yourself the foods that you really need, every single meal, every single day. This isn't about the rest of your life. It's about the *best* of your life.

DAY 22 MENU

▶ Breakfast

Popeye Smoothie

BLEND THE FOLLOWING INGREDIENTS UNTIL SMOOTH:

1 handful of spinach

1 frozen banana

1 tbsp. almond butter

2 scoops 22 Days plant-based protein powder

2 cups almond milk

▶ Lunch

Raw Zucchini, Carrot, and Cucumber Salad

INGREDIENTS:

1 zucchini

1 carrot

1 cucumber

1 tbsp. tahini

3 tbsp. lemon juice

dash sea salt

dash sesame seeds

1. Spiralize the zucchini, carrot, and cucumber.

2. Whisk together tahini, lemon juice, and sea salt.

3. In a mixing bowl, toss spiralized veggies with dressing.

4. Serve and top with sesame seeds.

▶ **Dinner**

Beluga Lentil Salad

INGREDIENTS:

1 cup beluga lentils

1 shallot

1 tbsp. lemon juice

1 tsp. apple cider vinegar

1 tsp. sea salt

½ tbsp. coriander

½ tbsp. cumin

1 tbsp. capers

2 tbsp. red pepper, diced

1 handful of fresh greens

1. Rinse the lentils and place them in a pot with 2 cups of water with sea salt, coriander, and cumin. Bring to a boil and simmer until desired tenderness is reached (15–20 minutes).

2. In a mixing bowl, combine the lentils with lemon, vinegar, capers, shallots, and pepper.

3. Arrange lentils over a bed of greens and top with lemon juice and vinegar.

EXERCISE

■ **RESISTANCE TRAINING:** Complete the exercises outlined on page 222.

MAINTAINING YOUR REVOLUTION

You've made it—and if you want to continue building up those benefits, keep it up. Even if you don't follow the menus precisely, you've developed a set of skills that can help you keep eating well. You learned to make plants a habit. You developed attention to consistency. You manifested a sense of awareness. You learned to eat with restraint.

Now what?

- Continue to eat plants—if what you're eating can't go bad, don't eat it!
- Use slipups as learning experiences instead of invitations to keep on slipping.
- Eat breakfast, lunch, and dinner instead of eating for emotional reasons.
- Give your food attention by sitting while you eat and eating slowly.
- Keep your home stocked with fresh fruits and vegetables instead of bulk processed foods.
- Prepare your meals and snacks in advance to make sure that healthy foods are just as fast as "fast foods."
- Eat right when you wake up in the morning, not right before you go to sleep at night.
- Refer to Chapter 18, "More Revolution Meals," to prepare tasty and tantalizing dishes you and everyone you love can enjoy—and thrive on!
- Remember that alcohol calories are empty calories, so choose them wisely. If you're going to reintroduce wine, do so with moderation and realize that it affects your weight and your health.

PART FOUR

POWER UP YOUR REVOLUTION:

Making the Program Work for You

13

MANAGE CHALLENGES
WITH GRACE

CHANGE ISN'T EASY. NOBODY SAID it was! If you want to make a real shift and get real benefits, you have to stick to the program in real time. And that includes challenges of all types—the ones that come from within, the ones that come from your physical environment, and the ones that come from what your friends and family are doing.

I'm here to tell you that it is possible! You can go to parties. You can go to restaurants. You can learn how to use challenges as opportunities to learn—even if you slip up! Every meal is an opportunity to eat plants. Every experience is a chance to learn so you can slowly, carefully, purposely make better choices that are going to get you exactly where you want to be.

PLANT-BASED PARTYING

As soon as you decide to make a change, lose weight, and get healthy, you know what happens: The invitations start coming in. Ten bar mitzvahs, two weddings, a birthday. Or holidays. Celebrations come up just when you've set your resolve to make a change. That's just the way life is. And I say to people, "You know what? Your will is being tested."

You've got to commit to the program fully no matter what events are on your social calendar! Events are all about people celebrating their lives. Why should someone else's celebration derail your careful plans to change and grow? Nobody wants that! And you don't have to make a choice—you can go to parties and enjoy yourself as long as you set yourself up for success.

Going to parties and sticking to your plant-based eating plan is all about strategy, just like most things. If you're invited to a wedding or a dinner where there is going to be an excess of tempting foods—do not go there hungry! Have a healthy snack at home to get yourself ready. When you arrive, look around and see what the healthiest foods are available, and you eat those.

And remember! You aren't there for the food. You're there for the people, for the socializing, for the dancing. So get out there and have a great time partying instead of eating.

If you're going to an event at a friend's home, a more casual event, call her in advance to get a sense of the menu. And offer to bring a healthy dish that you know fits into your new plant-based diet.

When you show up at the party with your platter of hummus and veggies, keep your eyes on it. Once you put it out, people will eat that quicker than they will eat potato chips. People want an excuse to eat healthy. They just want it to be convenient.

BRING THE REVOLUTION TO RESTAURANTS

You can bring food to share at a friend's house . . . but restaurants prefer that you stick to their menus. If you're going out to eat, there are some simple things you can do to make sure your meal is going to make you feel great instead of regretful.

- Call ahead or check out the menu online so that you can get your questions out of the way before you arrive.
- Don't go when you're starving! Ordering with hungry eyes leads to that awful overstuffed feeling later.
- Look for healthy, clean food. Things that are made of vegetables, as close to the earth as possible: fresh salads, vegetable

side dishes that are cooked or steamed lightly, vegetable soups, brown rice.

- Order salad dressing on the side and add it to taste, or get oil and vinegar and add it yourself.
- Stay away from white flour and white sugar.
- Say no to fried foods.
- Order fresh fruit for dessert.

EVERY SLIPUP IS AN OPPORTUNITY TO LEARN

Have you ever been walking down the sidewalk and suddenly your foot catches the edge of a crack and you stumble forward just a little bit? Just because you stumbled, you don't throw yourself to the ground. You say, "Whoa." And you look around to see whether anybody is looking, and they rarely are, and you think, *I feel foolish, but I'm good.* And you keep walking. It was just a little bump!

Same goes for diets. If you slip up, if your resolve wavers for a moment, you just dust yourself off and keep going, back on the plan.

Life is not *a reality TV show,* where you get sequestered into a ranch, and you get hand-fed nutritious foods like a baby bird. Life is like an all-you-can-eat buffet where you have to learn to keep your hands in your pockets if you can't keep them out of the bread pudding.

If you want to really rock the program, from 22 days to every single day, you've got to be ready to live in the real world, where challenges are frequent because unhealthy food abounds. Slipups are bound to happen, and when they do—use them, don't lose it.

A slipup is an opportunity to learn something about yourself, about what triggers you, and for you to fine-tune your strategies for success. So is a close call! If you almost, almost, almost eat the brownies, if you go back five times but then leave them alone—congratulations! You still need to think about what triggered that close call and how you can avoid it next time.

Once you know how to handle all of these situations, once you know how to navigate through these obstacles that life throws you, that is when you truly can find success. You will find success when you can truly navigate the course.

GIVE YOURSELF THE RIGHT REWARDS

Of course, navigating isn't only about going out. Sometimes it's about what happens when you get home.

I have a friend who lives in Los Angeles who has just about everything—on the surface. He has a thriving business, plenty of money, and a gorgeous home with incredible city views. This is a man who has achieved every kind of success, the kind of man other people are envious of, but because of our relationship I knew that he still felt unfulfilled.

For twenty years, he had been struggling with his weight. It was literally weighing him down. The extra forty pounds that he was carrying around were making him miserable, casting a shadow over all of his accomplishments. No matter what he did, no matter how much weight he managed to lose on one diet or another, he always found himself back at the same spot: overweight and unhappy.

What we realized after he did a lot of introspection and we talked his habits through was that he had no issues eating healthfully throughout the day. Breakfast, lunch, fantastic. But by the time he got home in the evenings, after what were usually very long and stressful days, he would feel like he deserved a reward for making it through the day.

Treating ourselves is a very good thing—when the reward is good for us. If he had indulged himself with a run or a massage, all would have been right with his world. But instead he gave himself with what he thought was a reward: food. If you look more closely, that chewy brownie every night wasn't really a reward—because after the first 30 seconds of pleasure while he was chewing, guilt and remorse set in.

First he felt guilty for having the brownie, because he was doing the one thing he really didn't want to do, which was eating foods that were making him unhealthy, which made him feel bad about himself. He was in a situation where he was perpetuating the feelings over and over again that he did not want to feel.

We talked it out.

"Why are you doing that?"

"Well, I'm hungry."

"You're not really hungry. You're coming home and you don't want to go straight to bed."

What we realized was that he wanted time to visualize his day. He wanted to run through the whole day again, thinking about what he did right and what he did wrong, what he could have done better. And then he wanted to unwind and relax, mellow down before getting in bed. In order to relax, he would turn to food, which was completely sabotaging him.

I said, "Why not find a better way to do that? Why not pick a great book? Why not find a little spot in your house and meditate? Why not sift through your thoughts quietly?"

And he really heard me. He said, "You know, I never really thought of it like that. You're right. I'm not really hungry. I don't even know why I'm eating. Half the time I don't even know what I eat. If you asked me what I ate last night I wouldn't know what to tell you."

I said, "That's how you know it's not a reward."

Rewards are special! Rewards are something we remember! If you can forget what you ate, it isn't really a reward.

What my friend realized was that he needed a better indulgence, something that would truly reward him instead of actually punishing him. He needed a better ritual for when he got home.

After a long conversation, he decided that instead of eating to relax, he would give himself what he needed: more sleep. So when he got home, instead of eating, he would wash his face and look in the mirror and say, "I did it. Another great day." And then he'd go to bed.

A week later he called me, so excited, and told me that it was working. He had finally given himself the right reward—and in the end, he knew it was the right kind of reward because it worked. It made him feel amazing. And that is what a reward is supposed to do.

So as you look more closely at your habits, at your reward system, at the ways you react to stress or a long day, or the way you celebrate, make sure you are choosing rewards that are really rewards. Because a reward should make you feel *great*!

14

REVOLUTION FITNESS

WHEN I WAS A KID, my uncle Paul was really fit. He was a cop, and the most muscular guy I knew, with these monster biceps. He was also the first guy I ever saw lifting weights, which taught me the very important lesson that what you do and what your body looks like are related. His fitness was so inspirational to me! And he did more than inspire—he gave me a place to work out by encouraging me to join the local policeman's program for youths, which meant that when I was old enough, I could use their gym. He gave me inspiration and he gave me the tools. That made all the difference for me.

As I grew older, it was so important to me that I be a role model to my children like my uncle was to me. Because that's how it works. Everything we know, we learned somewhere. The more conscious we can be about who our role models are, or the kinds of role models we want to be, the clearer our priorities become.

Is there anyone in your life who has inspired you to grow and learn and become the amazing person you are? Is there anyone in your life whom you would be proud and honored to inspire?

There's just something about watching someone you know take on a different shape that reminds us that our habits have real consequences. If you've been someone who experiences side effects from your habits that you don't want, like extra weight or the beginnings of an illness that is reversible and preventable, take charge now! Pick a hero, or choose to be somebody's hero—whatever starts a fire in your soul that tells you that you can do this.

I was very athletic when I was a kid, and I discovered good nutrition at a young age, as I've told you. But I was also a skinny kid without a lot of role models for good health, and seeing my uncle's fitness showed me that it was possible. For me, the next step was figuring out how, and that came from books as well as from the instruction I got at the gym.

I started doing sit-ups and push-ups. I started to use weights. I began to get stronger. And my friends noticed!

I remember waiting anxiously for the President's Challenge in school, an annual physical fitness challenge in schools across the country. I had my eyes on the prize—the Presidential Physical Fitness Award, that is. And I'd spend the year practicing my push-ups, pull-ups, and dips, and the consistency paid off every year.

It didn't take long before I became the expert on fitness among my friends. I showed them how to do push-ups, and I answered questions from the ones the adults called "husky" about how they could lose weight.

This was my personal discovery that I loved being someone who could share knowledge with people that could help them, and I resolved to learn as much as I could.

MAKE TIME INSTEAD OF EXCUSES

Do you make time to work out? Or do you create a list of excuses why you can't/don't have time? "Busy" isn't a reason not to work out!

I have a client named Frank who is a forty-something-year-old businessman. After years of neglecting his health and body, Frank decided that he would give plant-based a try, because he had seen firsthand that his brother had experienced great success with it. Frank was the kind of guy who lived to work; it was where he spent all of his time and energy. It soon became clear that Frank believed that if he went to the gym or spent any time doing anything pleasurable for himself during daylight or evening hours, he would sacrifice productivity—and for Frank, productivity was everything.

Just this one time, Frank agreed to go all in. Even though he was "too busy" and needed to "be productive," he promised that he would not just eat plants but also exercise. And Frank really did what he said he would do. He gave 100 percent. He dove in headfirst and immediately began an exercise program with a trainer at his local gym.

Can you guess what happened? Results happened, and Frank was hooked. By the twenty-second day he had lost 15 pounds and looked and felt better than he had in years.

The kicker was that he learned that his habit of just-work-no-fitness was not actually delivering maximum productivity. Frank turned out to be much more productive on a plant-based diet and a healthy, active workout schedule. New lifestyle, new health style, a more successful business. Because time spent on health is always time worth spending.

WHY EXERCISE MATTERS

There are so many good reasons for exercising that I could spend all day telling you about them. Except that I don't want you to sit here just learning about the value of exercise . . . I want you to get up and actually do it! So let's get a quick overview of some of the incredible benefits, and then you're going to put your sneakers on and get outside into the fresh air to help your body take advantage of all the amazing nutrition you've been giving yourself.

Exercise will help you:

- Lose weight, gain confidence, feel sexier. With more energy, that healthy glow, improved mood—suddenly everything about you is sexier. And you'll feel great about yourself too as your muscles become more shapely and the pounds keep falling off!
- Prevent disease and manage symptoms. High blood pressure, depression, stroke, some types of cancer, arthritis—being fit helps prevent a whole host of diseases, and can help you manage the symptoms of conditions you already have.
- Keep your heart healthy. People who are more active or more fit get less coronary heart disease . . . and if they do get it, it comes at a later age and is less severe.[65]

---

[65] http://circ.ahajournals.org/content/107/1/e2.full, accessed July 1, 2014.

- Get happier. Get rid of stress, raise your endorphin levels, ease depression, and give yourself a confidence boost: If you want to turn that frown upside down, get moving and get happy!
- Chill out. Who says you have to lie down to relax? Exercise can be one of the most efficient and beneficial ways to calm the mind and body, as well as offering a host of other benefits that will totally rock your revolution. If you're used to relaxing on the couch, start relaxing on the treadmill, in a yoga class or on a paddleboard instead, and just see how much more energy you have all day. When you work out, your heart pumps faster, your blood flows more efficiently, and more oxygen and more of the vitamins and minerals you eat can get where they need to go. And a stronger heart and lungs keep you jogging up those stairs no matter how many more flights there are to go, or how many grocery bags full of fresh veggies you're hauling.
- Keep your bones healthy. As we age, we can lose bone mass. Getting plenty of fitness, especially weight-bearing exercises, helps your bones stay strong so you can avoid diseases like osteoporosis.
- Lose the weight for good. Your fitness is the pillar that will support your plant-based diet so that you can lose that weight and keep it off. If you're here because you want to be leaner and thinner, working out will help you reach your goal. If you're here because you want to stay in the shape you're in, exercise can help you avoid weight gain. The more intense you get, the more you challenge yourself, the greater your personal results will be![66]

THE 22-DAY REVOLUTION WORKOUT

Fitness counts. If you want to achieve the best results, pay attention to your fitness. Just like plants need water plus sunlight to grow, human beings need a healthy balance in order to grow and flourish: We need

[66] http://www.mayoclinic.org/healthy-living/fitness/in-depth/exercise/art-20048389, accessed June 24, 2014.

the right foods and the right exercise, and we need to work at both. If you want real results you can't just do one thing—it's not diet or exercise; it's diet *and* exercise. There is no quick fix. Anybody who is promising you a quick fix or a shortcut is telling you something that isn't true.

I don't care if you use your body weight or the most high-tech equipment in the world. I've seen people transform their bodies using minimal equipment, and I've seen people work with the most high-tech equipment and remain the same over the years. . . . *Real success takes real hard work.* The key to success is consistency!

THE 22-DAY EXERCISE ROUTINE

CARDIO: Odd-numbered days are for cardio.

- Do 30–45 minutes of cardio followed by a 10–15-minute stretch.

RESISTANCE TRAINING: Even-numbered days are for resistance training.

- *Beginner:* 10 repetitions of exercises 1–7 (3x)
- *Intermediate:* 15 repetitions of exercises 1–7 (4x)
- *Advanced:* 25 repetitions of exercises 1–7 (4x)
- *Challenge me:* 100 burpees, 200 squats, 300 push-ups, 4 (one-minute) planks all in the shortest amount of time and then try to improve your time the next time you try it.

Cardio

When it comes to cardio, I advocate for at least 30–45 minutes three times a week. Cardio increases the workload of the heart and lungs, making them both more efficient. This kind of training will reduce risk of disease, improve heart function, and build stronger lungs and muscles, and ultimately you will be able to go harder and farther and faster than you ever imagined.

When you do your cardio, work at a pace at which a conversation would be difficult. Cardio helps you burn energy and raise your metabolism, as well improving your heart and lung function. By pacing yourself to work up a sweat, by challenging your heart and lungs, you'll know you are working effectively.

Some effective ways to get your cardio in and have some fun:

- Walking
- Jogging
- Running
- Sprints
- Jumping rope
- Cycling
- Swimming
- Rowing

Extra challenge: Check your timing! Completing a set course in a shorter amount of time is a great way to really feel the burn and work toward a goal.

Resistance

I've always been a fan of body-weight exercises, ever since my early days aiming for the Presidential Physical Fitness Award. The exercises suggested for your resistance training are simple and easy to follow, and no equipment should be needed. That's right! You don't need a gym membership. You don't need to go out and buy special, overpriced equipment. You just need the will to change!

For the next 22 days we'll use a simple, low-tech routine. While doing your moves, pay attention to your breathing: You'll want to breathe in during the eccentric (easy) part of the movement and breathe out during the concentric (difficult) part.

Focus on turning this series into a habit—while still remaining aware that you are doing the best thing possible for your body and your health by being consistent.

The following is a list of my favorite body-weight exercises:

1.

BURPEES

A burpee is a full-body aerobic exercise that moves you from standing to squatting to a push-up to a squat and back to standing. This should be done with as fluid a motion as possible, and should really warm you up.

The basic movement is performed in five steps:

1. Begin in a standing position.

2. Drop into a squat position and place your hands on the ground.

3. Kick your feet back, while keeping your arms extended.

4. Jump back into squat position with hands on the floor.

5. Jump up from the squat position while reaching for the sky with your hands.

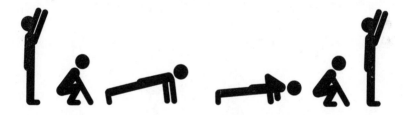

2.

SPLIT SQUATS

One of my favorite lower-body exercises. The split squat targets the quadriceps, hamstrings, glutes, and core. In addition, it builds balance and stability.

1. Position yourself into a staggered stance with your rear foot elevated on a bench or box and your front leg extended forward with foot firmly planted on the ground.

2. Slowly lower your body (making sure that your front foot is far enough in front of you so that your front knee remains over the ankle at the bottom of the movement) until the front thigh is parallel to the ground.

3. At the bottom of the movement, drive your hips forward and up as you press down on your heel to return to the start position.

▶ **TIP:** *Keep your back straight throughout the movement.*

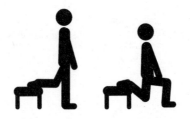

SQUATS

A compound, full-body exercise that works primarily the muscles of the thighs, as well as the glutes, hamstrings, hips, and core. The movement is simple but must be done properly to avoid injury and maximize results. Squats are amazing for building powerful thighs and legs. Move with purpose, and don't let gravity do the work for you!

1. Begin with feet firmly planted shoulder width apart (arms should be bent at 90 degrees and in front of the body for the entire movement).

2. Inhale as you drop your hips until your thigh is parallel to the ground while keeping your back straight.

3. Exhale and drive your hips forward as you lift and return to start position.

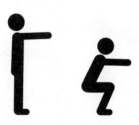

4.
PUSH-UPS

The push-up is one of the most common body-weight (calisthenic) exercises and is also used as an indicator of overall fitness. The push-up works the muscles of the chest, along with the triceps, shoulders, core, and serratus anterior, and develops muscular endurance.

1. Begin in a plank position (hands and feet placed shoulder width apart firmly on the ground with a straight line down the body).

2. Inhale as you bend at the elbow and drop down until the chest touches the ground (lightly).

3. Exhale as you press and lift your upper body back to starting position.

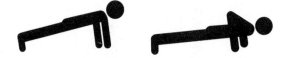

5.
REVERSE DIPS

Reverse dips have long held their place in gyms across the world because of the benefits this simple move yields. Muscles worked are the triceps, and those in the shoulders, back, and neck. Reverse dips are great for defining the back of the arm and sculpting shoulders!

1. Begin with your arms fully extended and hands firmly placed on a bench behind you.

2. Extend your legs straight out in front of you (or on another bench for added difficulty).

3. Begin to bend at the elbow as you lower your body past the bench until the upper arm is parallel to the ground.

4. Squeeze your triceps and lift your body back to start position with arms fully extended.

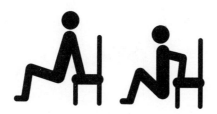

6.
PLANKS

The plank is great for building the muscles of the core in addition to building balance and muscular endurance.

1. Begin in a push-up position with arms fully extended and a straight line down the body.

2. Hold position (30 seconds) by flexing the muscles of the core and arms.

▶ **BEGINNER MODIFICATION:** *Feel free to try this move on your elbows as well.*

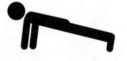

SIDE PLANK

The side plank, like the plank, is great for building the muscles of the core, with an added emphasis on balance and muscular endurance.

1. Lie on your side with your legs straight and fully extended.

2. Prop up your body with the arm closest to the ground fully extended under your shoulder.

3. Raise your hips until your body forms a straight line down to your ankles.

4. Hold this position (30 seconds).

5. Repeat on opposite side.

▶ **BEGINNER MODIFICATION:** *Feel free to try this move on your elbows as well.*

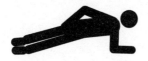

Challenge yourself! How long did it take you to complete your routine? Next time, try to shave off a few minutes. I often use this routine with clients, and for an added challenge I will set a timer to really make them work!

Want a bigger challenge? Do 100 burpees, 200 squats, 300 push-ups, and 4 (one-minute) planks. How quickly can you finish the challenge? Best it the next time you try it!

USE PLANT PROTEIN TO BUILD MUSCLE

NUTRITION AND FITNESS go close in hand when it comes to health. Carbohydrates and fat provide energy, and if you're looking for maximum muscle, you'll get everything you need from plant protein!

I work with a lot of guys who worry about where their protein is going to come from. Trust me, there is plenty of protein found in a balanced, plant-based diet, and it's much better for muscle building than animal protein. When we exercise, we create inflammation in our muscles. When you're in the recovery process, your body wants to reduce that inflammation so that you can accelerate the recovery phase.

Eating meat actually exacerbates the inflammation.[67] It's too taxing to your body. But a plant-based diet helps your body repair without the inflammation. A study compared head-to-head whey protein and rice protein—and in terms of muscle gain, the effects were no different between using whey protein and rice protein.[68]

If you really, truly want to build good, strong muscles, you should consume more plant-based foods, so that you can minimize the inflammation of the body. Because the quicker you minimize inflammation, the faster the recovery—and the quicker you can get into another workout.

That's why many athletes, like triathletes and Ironmen who sign up for really long, grueling races, choose plant-based foods as an incredible source for maximum workout power.

When I worked with Robert, he was a full-time student and an aspiring professional triathlete. Robert was looking for an edge and decided to give the 22-Day Revolution program a try. Within a day, his digestion improved. He slept better that night, too. That made him think he might be onto something special! Within a week, Robert was experiencing shorter recovery times after his workouts and sustained energy during his longer workouts. By the twenty-second day, he decided he had to share this lifestyle with his family and all his friends (except the ones who raced against him).

[67] http://www.ncbi.nlm.nih.gov/pubmed/24284436, accessed June 25, 2014.

[68] http://www.nutritionj.com/content/12/1/86, accessed June 25, 2014.

THE 22-DAY REVOLUTION VACATION

Don't take a vacation from your revolution: Take it on vacation with you! Going on vacation does not mean you have an all-access pass to indulge and forgo exercise. In fact, it's quite the opposite. Vacation gives you the time and space to reset and relax. So focus on your habits and getting back to basics while you're away. It's also a great time to try some new kinds of exercise on a fitness-related vacation. Think about it—you love working out, so why not incorporate fun fitness activities into a vacation?

It can help to put some forethought into choosing your destination by looking at each one and its access to fitness. You can also tailor your destination to suit your fitness needs, such as choosing a location with access to running or bike trails, or a resort with yoga classes.

CHOOSE A HOTEL WITH FITNESS OPTIONS. If you're traveling for business or pleasure, choose a resort or hotel that caters to active people so you can get moving while you're on the move. Many places offer a gym, yoga, and bike rentals.

CHECK OUT A NATIONAL PARK. If you're into hiking, biking, and other activities and you're a self-starter, there are parks across the country just waiting for you to explore. In the United States, you can even buy a National Parks Passport that will make it fun for your family to rack up the stamps every time you visit a new national park.

GO FOR A BIKE RIDE. Biking enthusiasts can enjoy amazing vacations biking along the many Rails-to-Trails pathways in the U.S. The Web site can help you map out your daily distances and find lodging in quaint towns along the way: http://www. railstotrails.org /

LEARN SOMETHING NEW. Have you ever tried stand-up paddleboarding, surfing, diving, yoga, tennis? These activities combine fitness and fun. And if you're ready for an active new hobby, committing to a full week or more of the activity will make you a pro in no time.

VACATION WITH AN ACTIVE TOUR GROUP. Instead of a cruise, if you love tours, choose one that is as interested in sports as you are. There are bike tours, yoga retreats, hiking tours, or scuba diving trips; look for a tour group that can offer you a multiday excursion. There's a tour for pretty much every activity to meet most budgets. Not only will you have a great time, but by committing to your activity for an extended period of time you'll up your game and come back even more fit than ever.

15

FAST-TRACK YOUR WEIGHT LOSS

EVERY PERSON ON THE PLANET can benefit from a plant-based diet: if you are at a healthy body weight, as I was when I shifted to plant-based living, you still get the health benefits from eating plants. For people who have more than thirty pounds to lose, the fast-track program will help you lose weight and overhaul those unhealthy habits. Eating plants is the best way to get that weight off and *keep it off.*

Before we get started, I'd like to look at some definitions about weight. We hear the words *overweight* and *obese* often, so let's clarify. According to the CDC, if you are overweight, you have too much weight for your height, and that weight comes from fat, muscle, bone, water, or a combination. If you are obese, you have excess body fat. Both being overweight and being obese come from eating too much food. If you are overweight and/or obese, you have been eating more calories at meals and snacks than you have been burning with your daily activities, probably for a long time.

If you want to lose weight, you must take in fewer calories and burn more calories—probably for a long time. In a world that demands immediate results, the idea that real change takes real time can be scary. But if you want real and lasting change, I'm here to tell you that *it is possible*—as long as you commit.

The fast track works by teaching you to eat less and encouraging you to engage in fitness more. It's important to understand that weight is gained one pound at a time, and that's also how it's lost: pound by pound by pound. The more weight you have put on over the years, the longer it will take to get those pounds off of your body. Extreme weight loss takes commitment! When you have thirty or fifty or even one hundred pounds to lose, you know up-front that it's going to be a long road. That's why I invite you to really commit. To really go the distance, you need to embrace the hard work required to reach your goal and then give the program all you've got.

The harder you work, the more commitment you have, the faster you'll get there—and the more likely that you'll keep going.

We're very conditioned to pay attention to risk versus reward. If we risk something—for instance, if we decide to make a big change in our lives that requires a lot of energy and consciousness—we want to know that we're going to be rewarded. So if you decide to lose fifty pounds, and you spend a week or two eating in a completely different style, the faster the weight comes off, the more motivated you're going to be to keep that change going. The more motivated you're going to be to stay committed.

If you have upward of 30 pounds to lose, you need to commit 100 percent. When you have five or ten pounds to lose, even if you're losing only a pound or two a week, you're going to get there quickly. Losing more weight takes more time, and it takes more effort. But the payoff is *tremendous*. The boost of energy that you'll get, the boost of confidence that you'll earn—trust me. It's going to be worth it.

That's why the fast-track program requires your complete participation. I want you to see results so you stay motivated. I don't want you to work hard for two weeks and then be disillusioned because the results aren't aggressive enough for you.

If you want big results, make a big commitment.

HOW TO FAST-TRACK

Fast-Track Your Menus

- **Meal replacement.** If you want to challenge yourself even more, or if you have more than 30 pounds to lose, replace dinner or breakfast with a smoothie a few times per week (check out the recipes for my favorite combinations in Chapter 18). Why dinner or breakfast? In my experience, lunch is a meal that most people can stick to. At lunchtime, we're all usually very conscious of what we're eating and at our best for adhering to healthy guidelines. Meanwhile, dinner is the one meal where people usually overindulge. And breakfast is the meal that people usually skip, putting themselves in a terrible position for lunch and dinner.

As a meal replacement, try a 22-Days Nutrition protein powder in one of the smoothies, or try a 22-Days bar as an easy grab-and-go meal. Both pack an incredible amount of protein in delicious and satisfying flavors that will supercharge your weight loss. If you're going to fast-track, decide whether you're replacing dinner or breakfast and then stick with the plan!

For a more aggressive approach, or if you have more than 50 pounds to lose, supercharge your weight loss even more by replacing your dinner with a green juice at least four times per week. Start your day with a smoothie for breakfast, and lunch from the meal plan, and then whip up your favorite green juice at night. Add a 30–45 minute cardio workout, and you'll see incredible results of up to 1 pound per day.

- **Carb shift.** As you know by now, the 22-days program is about embracing carbs and aiming for an 80-10-10 breakdown of carbohydrates, protein, and fat. If your goal is to lose a significant amount of weight, shift the meals and eat the denser, more carb-heavy option for lunch instead of dinner. Your body will use its own resources (fat stores!) for digestion and repair overnight, instead of the carb-based fuel you normally eat at dinnertime.

- **Intermittent fasting.** Have more than 50 pounds to lose? Try intermittent fasting.[69] Whether it's skipping meals every once in a while or every other day, we practice it already and don't even know it. It's called sleeping; hence your first meal of the day is called break-*fast*. Intermittent fasting just gets you to extend the

---

[69] http://www.independent.ie/life/health-wellbeing/health-features/the-fast-way-to-lose-weight-live-healthily-and-fight-ageing-30605034.html, accessed October 13, 2014.

fasting period. For more than 80 years doctors and scientists have been exploring the benefits of reducing calories by skipping meals. In short, don't be afraid to skip a meal here and there if you're up to the added challenge and increased benefits the reduced caloric intake may offer. Check with your doctor before beginning this or any other weight loss program.

Fast-Track Your Fitness

- **Cardio.** To increase your weight loss, you must increase exercise. Use the fitness chapter to the best of your ability. Make sure to engage in sweat-inducing cardio for 45–60 minutes six days a week, even if it's just a brisk walk.

- **Make a plan and stick to it.** One of the most common struggles my clients have with working out is finding the time in their busy schedules to get to the gym consistently. I personally love workouts in the morning, because it's the one time of the day you can stick to by just getting up earlier, whereas afternoon or night workouts can easily get derailed by busy lives and hectic work schedules. If you want to be consistent and have been struggling to find the time, it's simple: Wake up an hour earlier.

- **Intensity matters.** The best way to see results quickly is to make your workouts fast and explosive. Short, intense workouts have been found to yield the greatest results. So get your workouts done quickly by taking fewer breaks and by doing exercises that combine multiple muscle groups, like the moves suggested in the Revolution Fitness chapter (page 217).

PART FIVE

REVOLUTION FOR LIFE:

Recipes and Motivation for Day 23 and Beyond

16

AFTER 22 DAYS

ONCE YOU'RE ACCUSTOMED TO EATING food from the earth, dieting is something you'll no longer need to think about. The hard work on this program is changing your habits from unconsciously eating processed food throughout the day to mindfully eating plant-based meals. Once plants are your habit, the journey is easy! That's because nature knows best. Plant-based food is perfectly designed to sustain us. When you follow the daily menus on this program, you don't have to count calories or macronutrients, because the right balance is built into the menus. That will train your body to become accustomed to how it really feels to eat the right foods.

After completing the program, you'll be ready to take it to the next level—and you still won't have to count calories or macronutrients. Once you know your habits are transformed, eating a variety of plants will naturally give you the healthy balance of 80-10-10, and listening to your internal cues will keep you from eating too much at mealtimes. Sustainable weight loss will be inevitable!

You have the power to customize the menus to make the program work for you. Some people become plant-based eaters for the long haul, because they want to keep getting those benefits day after day. Some people adjust back into eating fish or lean protein along with their plants. Some people use the challenge as a reset anytime they just want to feel great!

FOR A BETTER RESULT, MAKE BETTER CHOICES

How many people do you know who lose ten pounds ten times during the year? That kind of up and down indicates there's something unsustainable about their approach. The goal isn't to lose ten pounds again and again—the goal is to create the habits that'll help you get there—and stay there. You've spent 22 days eating the best food the planet has to offer, and today you're going to make a choice about what to do tomorrow.

Do you want results that stick? Or do you want to revert back to the way things used to be?

Einstein brilliantly said that the definition of insanity is doing the same thing over and over again and expecting different results. Why haven't your past diets made an impact? Why does yo-yo dieting happen? Because you keep doing the same thing. You get on and you get off. Of course it isn't going to work. Every set of actions has a result. Did the old way work for you? If the answer is no, you owe it to yourself to find a better way.

This time, try a different way. Embrace your new healthy habits and stick with the program so that you make them permanent, and see those sustainable results. And when you feel that inner urge to veer off the right path, you're going to notice right away, because you're now in tune with your body and needs. You're going to say, "Here is the spot where I used to make a wrong turn, every time."

And then you're going to stay in your lane, because health and happiness are just up ahead.

17

SUBLIME SMOOTHIES

SMOOTHIES MAKE A GREAT BREAKFAST, and they are a perfect meal replacement whether you're trying to fast-track your weight loss (see Chapter 15 for details) or eating plant-based to maintain a healthy weight for the long-term.

For each, combine all the ingredients in a blender and blend until smooth.

Lean Green Smoothie

4 stalks of kale

1 handful of spinach

1 frozen banana

2 green apples

1 lemon (juiced)

Popeye Protein Smoothie

1 handful of spinach

1 frozen banana

1 tbsp. almond butter

2 scoops of 22 Days plant-based protein powder

2 cups of almond milk

Jungle Gym

2 scoops 22 Days plant-based protein powder (chocolate)

2 cups almond milk

1 frozen banana

Recover and Repair

2 scoops 22 Days plant-based protein powder (vanilla)

2 cups coconut water

1 cup frozen blueberries

▲ 1 tbsp. flaxseed oil

Green Machine

2 scoops 22 Days plant-based protein powder (vanilla)

1 handful kale

1 handful spinach

1 frozen banana

3 pitted dates

2 cups almond milk

Chocolate Dream

2 scoops 22 Days plant-based protein powder (chocolate)

2 cups almond milk (chocolate)

1 tbsp. almond butter

1 cup ice

Green Awareness

2 scoops 22 Days plant-based protein powder (vanilla)

2 cups almond milk

1 handful spinach

1 frozen banana

1 tbsp. almond butter

Tropical Power

2 scoops 22 Days plant-based protein powder (vanilla)

2 cups almond milk

½ cup frozen mango

½ cup frozen peaches

S'mores

2 scoops 22 Days plant-based protein powder (chocolate)

2 cups almond milk

6 vegan graham crackers (or ½ cup homemade granola)

1 frozen banana

Orange Creamsicle

2 scoops 22 Days plant-based protein powder (vanilla)

2 cups vanilla almond milk

½ frozen orange

1 frozen banana

Peanut Butter Banana

2 scoops 22 Days plant-based protein powder (vanilla or chocolate)

2 cups almond milk

1 frozen banana

2 small pitted dates

1 tbsp. peanut butter

1 tbsp. chia seeds

Imagination Creation

2 scoops 22 Days plant-based protein powder (chocolate or vanilla)

2 cups favorite milk substitute (water and coconut water included)

2 cups leafy greens

2 cups frozen fruit

On-the-Run Protein Smoothie

On the run? No problem. Pour into a travel cup and take with you for a protein-packed power punch.

2 scoops 22 Days plant-based protein powder (chocolate)

2 cups almond milk

1 frozen banana

1 tbsp. sunflower butter

18

MORE REVOLUTION MEALS

AFTER YOUR 22-DAY REVOLUTION, ONCE you've gotten into the habit of keeping your home stocked with fresh fruits and vegetables, once you've experienced how satisfying plant-based eating is, you'll want to keep on going. So we've put together a collection of our family classics to keep inspiring you in the kitchen, from hearty oatmeal to homemade almond milk, from sandwich fillings to a Thai twist on noodles.

Breakfast, lunch, dinner and snacks, eating plants tastes as good as it makes you feel. These recipes are some of my favorites, from my family cookbook to yours.

Chunky Cinnamon Apple Oatmeal

1 SERVING

INGREDIENTS:

½ cup dry oats

½ small Fuji apple, peeled and diced

⅔ cup almond milk

⅓ cup water

1 tbsp. almond butter

1 tsp. milled flax

▲ 4 almonds, chopped

dash cinnamon

1. In a small bowl, combine the almond milk, water, almond butter, chopped almonds and oats in a pot over medium-low heat. Bring to a simmer, stirring frequently.
2. Once oatmeal begins to thicken, add in the diced apple and stir a few times.
3. Remove from heat and serve.
4. Top with milled flax and a dash of cinnamon.

Muesli

8 SERVINGS

INGREDIENTS:

3⅔ cups gluten-free rolled oats

½ cup dried cranberries

⅓ cup golden raisins

⅓ cup sunflower seeds

▲ ⅓ cup pumpkin seeds

▲ ⅓ cup sliced almonds

¼ cup walnuts, chopped

▲ ¼ cup cashews, chopped

½ tsp. ground cinnamon

1. Preheat oven to 350 degrees.
2. Place oats on baking sheet and bake for 5 minutes or until golden brown.
3. Remove and cool completely.
4. In a large mixing bowl, mix together all the ingredients and store in an airtight container (Ball mason jars are great) until ready to eat.
▲ 5. Can be enjoyed with favorite nut drink and topped with fresh fruit and milled flaxseed.

Almond Milk

We use almond milk with tons of recipes at home, including with our oatmeal for breakfast. After trying all the commercial products available, I decided I'd try to make my own. Turns out I absolutely love it, and the process just feels right! Less waste, no unnecessary additives, less sugar, better for the planet, and most important . . . better for my kids, and they love it!

WHAT YOU'LL NEED:

Nut milk bag or cheesecloth
Blender
Large bowl

INGREDIENTS:

▲ 2 cups of raw almonds
7 cups water
2 large pitted medjool dates or 2 tbsp. organic maple syrup
1 whole vanilla bean (chopped) or 1 tsp. vanilla
1 pinch of fine-grain sea salt to enhance flavor

1. Place the raw almonds in a bowl, cover with water, and soak overnight (8–12 hours).
2. Rinse and drain the almonds and place them into the blender along with the rest of the ingredients (including water).
3. Blend on highest speed until smooth (usually about one and a half minutes).
4. Pour the mixture into nut milk bag while holding it over a bowl.
5. Gently squeeze the bag to release the milk and repeat until all the milk has been squeezed out.
6. Pour into glass jars and store in the refrigerator for up to five days. Mixture separates when sitting; shake well before using.
7. Don't be afraid to experiment until you discover your own perfect recipe!

Better Than Tuna Salad

INGREDIENTS:

- ▲ 1 cup raw almonds
  2 celery stalks
  1 garlic clove, finely chopped (optional)
  2 tbsp. vegan mayo
  1 tbsp. fresh lemon juice
  1 tsp. mustard
  1 dash sea salt
  1 dash fresh ground pepper

1. Soak almonds overnight in a bowl of water. Drain and rinse.
2. Place almonds into a food processor until finely chopped. Place into a mixing bowl.
3. Mix all the other ingredients together and toss until even mix is achieved.
4. Place mix over a bed of greens (spinach, kale, romaine) and enjoy.
5. Can also be enjoyed in a lettuce wrap or vegan bread of choice topped with tomatoes and avocado.

Buddha Bowl

2–3 SERVINGS

INGREDIENTS:

1 head of broccoli

1 head of cauliflower

2 kale leaves

1½ cups cooked chickpeas (or preferred bean)

1 cup cooked brown rice or quinoa

1 plum tomato

2 tbsp. tahini

1 lemon

1 tsp. nutritional yeast

salt and pepper, to taste

1. Lightly steam broccoli, cauliflower, and kale.
2. Place steamed veggies in a bowl and neatly place 1 serving of cooked grains next to it. Add the chickpeas and the tomato.
3. Drizzle tahini dressing (2 tbsp. of tahini mixed with the juice of 1 lemon) over the top and add salt, pepper and nutritional yeast to taste.

Veggie Pad Thai

2 SERVINGS

INGREDIENTS:

- 1 medium zucchini (spiraled)
- 2 large carrots (julienned)
- 1 red pepper (thinly sliced)
- 3 green onions (thinly sliced)
- 1 head of broccoli (steamed)
- 1 cup mung bean sprouts

DRESSING:

- 1 garlic clove chopped
- ¼ cup almond butter
- 1 lime
- 2 tbsp. coconut aminos (or low-sodium tamari)
- 2 tbsp. maple syrup
- 1 tsp. finely grated ginger
- 2 tbsp. water
- ½ tbsp. toasted sesame oil

- 1 tbsp. hulled hempseeds
- 1 tbsp. sesame seeds

1. Prepare vegetables as called for in ingredient list and add into large mixing bowl. Toss to combine.
2. Mix all dressing ingredients together in a food processor or by hand (whisking).
3. Top veggies with dressing and top with sesame and hempseeds.

Sautéed Zucchini with Pine Nuts and Basil

2–3 SERVINGS

INGREDIENTS:

3 large zucchini (sliced)

3 tbsp. pine nuts

½ tbsp. cold-pressed olive oil

4 fresh basil leaves

2 cloves of garlic (finely chopped)

1 tbsp. capers

1 tbsp. balsamic vinegar

salt and pepper, to taste

1. In a large skillet or pan heat a tablespoon of olive oil over medium heat. Add the zucchini and sauté until golden brown (you may have to do this twice to get all the zucchini).
2. In a large mixing bowl toss in all the other ingredients except 1 basil leaf you'll save for garnish.
3. Once all the zucchini is golden brown, toss together with your mix and place it back in the pan. Toss well for a minute or so and then move to serving plate.
4. Garnish with chopped basil. Add salt and pepper to taste.

Baked Chickpeas over Greens

2 SERVINGS

INGREDIENTS:

2 cups cooked chickpeas

2 tsp. coconut aminos

1 tbsp. balsamic vinegar

½ tsp. oregano

½ tsp. rosemary

½ tsp. maple syrup

3 cups of greens (of choice)

½ avocado, cubed

1 plum tomato

1. Preheat oven to 375 degrees.
2. Toss all ingredients together in a mixing bowl.
3. Place all the ingredients over a lined (parchment paper) baking sheet and bake for 20 minutes, tossing a few times throughout.
4. Remove when chickpeas are golden in color and almost dry.
5. Serve over a bed of greens and top with chopped avocado and tomato.

Aloo Gobi (Potato and Cauliflower Curry)

6 SERVINGS

INGREDIENTS:

1 head of cauliflower (cut into bite-size florets)

2 medium potatoes, cubed

1 onion, chopped

2 Roma tomatoes, chopped

2 tbsp. coconut oil

1 tsp. minced garlic

½ tsp. coriander

½ tsp. turmeric

1 tbsp. cumin

¼ tsp. ground ginger

¼ tsp. cinnamon

¼ tsp. cayenne pepper (or more to taste)

½ tsp. sea salt

1. Heat the oil in a medium skillet over medium heat.
2. Add in onion, garlic, coriander, turmeric, cumin, ground ginger, cinnamon, cayenne pepper, and sea salt.
3. Cook for 1 minute, or until onion is lightly browned.
4. Add the potatoes, cover, and cook for an additional 7–10 minutes.
5. Add cauliflower, reduce heat to low, and cover. Stir occasionally and cook for an additional 10 minutes, or until cauliflower and potatoes are tender.
6. Mix in diced tomato when ready to serve.

Raw Walnut Crumble in an Avocado Cup

4 SERVINGS

INGREDIENTS:

2 Haas avocados sliced in half (leave skin on)

WALNUT CRUMBLE:

2 cups walnuts

1½ tbsp. cumin

1 tbsp. coriander

2 tbsp. balsamic vinegar

1 tbsp. coconut aminos

dash paprika

dash garlic powder

dash black ground pepper

GARNISH INGREDIENTS:

½ pint cherry tomatoes (1 small pack)

½ tbsp. dried parsley flakes

pinch black ground pepper

pinch sea salt

1 lime

1. Combine all taco ingredients in a food processor.
2. Pulse several times until crumbly, making sure not to overblend.
3. Spread the walnut taco meat evenly over the avocado half (portion out enough taco meat to make 4 even servings).
4. Chop tomatoes and use as topping.
5. Garnish with parsley, ground pepper, sea salt, and lime juice.

Quinoa and Kidney Bean Salad

3–4 SERVINGS

INGREDIENTS:

- 1 cup quinoa
- 1 cup kidney beans
- 1 small red onion, finely chopped
- 1 tsp. cumin
- 1 tsp. coriander
- 1 carrot (julienned)
- ½ tsp. fine sea salt
- dash black ground pepper
- 2 lemons
- 2 tbsp. extra virgin olive oil

1. Rinse one cup of quinoa in a fine sieve, drain, and transfer to a medium pot.
2. Add 2 cups of water and a pinch of salt. Bring to a boil and simmer until the water is absorbed and quinoa is fluffy (15–20 minutes).
3. Toss (cooled) quinoa in a mixing bowl with the kidney beans, onion, and carrot.
4. In another bowl, whisk together lemon juice, olive oil, cumin, coriander, sea salt, and pepper.
5. Pour the dressing over the quinoa and toss to coat evenly.

Chickpea Hand Rolls

2–4 SERVINGS

INGREDIENTS:

1 head butter lettuce

1 cup cooked chickpeas (slightly mashed)

4 teaspoons tahini

2 lemons

1 teaspoon coconut aminos

½ tbsp. cumin

¼ cup diced celery

1 tbsp. parsley

sea salt and pepper to taste

1. Toss all the ingredients (except chickpeas and butter lettuce) in a mixing bowl and whisk until smooth.
2. Pour mix over chickpeas and toss to coat evenly.
3. Scoop chickpea mix onto lettuce cup and wrap neatly into a small hand roll.

Homemade Hummus

When we go to parties, we bring a hummus-and-veggie platter with us, and believe me—it's gone before the chips even have a chance. I'm not sure anyone realizes that the fresh, crunchy celery they're enjoying may be used to treat joint pain (rheumatism), is good for relaxation and sleep; has plenty of fiber to help keep you regular and may help control intestinal gas. The chemicals in celery may decrease symptoms of arthritis, as well as low blood pressure and blood sugar, and help muscles relax. And cucumber offers a host of benefits with every crisp bite. Now, that's a power party food![70]

INGREDIENTS:

1¾ cups chickpeas, cooked (15-ounce can), or see below for cooking instructions using 1 cup dry

¼ cup chickpea water (if using canned chickpeas, rinse and drain, setting aside ¼ cup of the liquid from can)

4 tbsp. lemon juice

1 tbsp. tahini

¼ tsp. sea salt, or to taste

pinch paprika

4 celery stalks

1 bunch baby carrots

1 large cucumber

DIRECTIONS FOR COOKING CHICKPEAS:

1. Presoak 1 cup chickpeas overnight in 4 cups of water to reduce cooking time, or quick-soak: Cover beans with water, bring to a boil for 2 minutes, then remove from heat and let sit for 1–2 hours.

2. Rinse, drain, then cover with 3 cups of fresh water and continue cooking.

3. Bring water and beans to a boil, reduce heat, cover, and let simmer, skimming off any foam and stirring occasionally (presoaked beans will take about 1 hour to cook).

---

[70] http://www.webmd.com/vitamins-supplements/ingredientmono-882-CELERY.aspx?activeIngredientId=882&activeIngredientName=CELERY, accessed July 22, 2014.

4. Beans are done when tender.

5. Rinse, drain, and let cool. (Makes about 2 cups cooked chickpeas.) Once chickpeas are cooled, store leftovers in fridge for a few days, or in freezer for up to 6 months.

DIRECTIONS FOR HUMMUS AND PLATTER:

1. Combine all ingredients in a blender or food processor, except the chickpea water.

2. Blend until thoroughly mixed and smooth, adding chickpea water 1 tbsp. at a time until desired consistency is reached.

3. Place in a serving bowl and sprinkle with a dash of paprika.

Marilyn's Carrot Bread with Frosting

I love to cook and prepare fresh foods for my family and friends, but I love it even more when my wife, Marilyn, and my boys join me. Marilyn is fascinating to watch, because she was born with a gift that gives her the ability to turn any food into an incredibly delicious and, of course, healthy dish you'll wish you had the recipe for.

INGREDIENTS:

1 cup unpacked finely grated carrot

¾ cup sweetened vanilla almond milk

½ cup maple syrup (add 1 additional tbsp. you if prefer sweeter)

1 tbsp. warm coconut oil, or canola oil (optional)

2 tbsp. applesauce

1 tsp. vanilla extract

½ tsp. apple cider vinegar

½ cup brown-rice flour

½ cup gluten-free oat flour

¼ cup tapioca flour

¼ cup arrowroot flour

½ cup almond flour

1 tbsp. flax meal

1 tbsp. ground chia seeds

2 tsp. baking powder

½ tsp. baking soda

1 tsp. ground cinnamon

⅛ tsp. sea salt

¼ cup walnuts, chopped (optional)

INGREDIENTS FOR FROSTING:

1 cup raw cashews, soaked, drained, and rinsed (or macadamia nuts)

1 tsp. lemon juice

2 tbsp. maple syrup (add more if you prefer sweeter)

¼ cup sweetened vanilla almond milk

DIRECTIONS FOR FROSTING:

1. In a blender or food processor, blend all ingredients until smooth, adding water as needed, and put in the refrigerator until ready to use.

DIRECTIONS:

1. Preheat oven to 350°F and lightly grease a small (8-inch-by-4-inch) loaf pan or 8-inch round cake pan.

2. In a bowl, mix together the almond milk, maple syrup, oil, applesauce, vanilla, and apple cider vinegar. Set aside while preparing the dry ingredients. If adding the coconut oil, make sure the wet ingredients are at room temperature to prevent the oil from hardening.

3. In another bowl, whisk together the gluten-free flour blend, almond flour, flax meal, chia seeds, baking powder, baking soda, cinnamon, and salt.

4. Pour the wet ingredients over the dry and stir until just combined. Then fold in the carrots and walnuts (or other nut of choice).

5. Pour into loaf pan lined with parchment paper and bake for about 50 minutes or until you can slide a knife into the center and it comes out clean. Remove pan from oven and let cool before transferring the loaf from pan to wire rack. Let cool completely (at last an hour), then slice and serve! Makes about 12 servings.

6. If baking in a cake pan, then bake for 40–45 minutes. Remove pan from oven and let cool before transferring the cake from the pan to a wire rack. Once completely cool, spread the frosting, slice, and enjoy. (To make a double-layered cake, simply double up the recipe and evenly divide the batter into two cake pans.)

7. If there are any leftovers (which is usually not the case in my house), store in an airtight container at room temperature for no more than a few days, in the refrigerator for up to a week, or in the freezer for no more than a few months. Slices should be individually wrapped with plastic freezer wrap or layered with parchment paper in freezer bags.

8. Enjoy a slice or two for breakfast or as a snack. This carrot bread is simple, healthy, nutritious, and delicious! For a lighter treat, have it without walnuts and save the frosting for special occasions. You can also explore using this recipe to make other variations. I've tried making carrot muffins with this batter instead of a cake or a loaf, or making a zucchini bread loaf by simply substituting the carrots with zucchini. Just be creative!

Marilyn's Hearty Multigrain Bread

How can a bread be this good and be gluten-free? Because there are a wealth of flours out there that are fabulous when combined in the right ratios. Here, we use Marilyn's special mixture of quinoa flour, brown-rice flour, gluten-free oat flour, and a few others . . . try it and see the difference!

INGREDIENTS:

1 cup water (warm)

2¼ tsp. dry active yeast

2 tsp. raw cane sugar

1 cup unsweetened almond milk (warm)

1 tbsp. canola oil (or high-heat safflower oil)

2 tsp. apple cider vinegar

▲ 1 cup quinoa flour

½ cup brown-rice flour

½ cup gluten-free oat flour

½ cup arrowroot flour

½ cup tapioca starch/flour

2 tbsp. almond flour

4 tbsp. ground chia seeds

1 tbsp. flax meal

1 tsp. baking powder

½ tsp. baking soda

½ tsp. salt

▲ 2 tbsp. pumpkin seeds (optional)

2 tbsp. sunflower seeds (optional)

DIRECTIONS:

1. In a bowl, combine the warm water with the yeast and sugar and allow it to froth for about 5–10 minutes. Then add the warm almond milk, oil, and apple cider vinegar and set aside.

2. In another bowl, combine all the dry ingredients and whisk well.

3. Pour the wet ingredients into the dry and stir well. Gently fold in the pumpkin and sunflower seeds or other seeds/nuts of choice.

4. Pour batter into a lined loaf pan (8 by 4 inches), using the back of a spoon to gently press and smooth out the top of the batter. You can also sprinkle gluten-free oats and/or seeds on top of the loaf.

5. Cover the loaf pan with a kitchen cloth or plastic wrap and set aside to allow the loaf to rise for approximately 45 minutes. Check on loaf after 30 minutes and remove towel or wrap to allow loaf to fully rise.

6. Preheat oven to 350°F.

7. Bake the loaf for about 50 minutes.

8. Remove pan from the oven and let cool before transferring the loaf from the pan to a wire rack. Let cool completely before slicing. There will be approximately 14 servings.

9. Store any leftovers in an airtight container at room temperature for no more than a few days, in the refrigerator for up to a week, or in the freezer for no more than 4 to 6 months. Slices should be individually wrapped with plastic freezer wrap or layered with parchment paper in freezer bags.

10. This hearty bread can be enjoyed any time of the day! Have it for breakfast toasted with almond butter or simply with a side of berries and fresh juice, or make a sandwich using your favorite ingredients, like avocado, hummus, or baked eggplant, or a veggie burger with tomato, lettuce, etc. Enjoy!

Marilyn's Mini Chocolate-Chip Muffins

The kids love these, and I love that they can enjoy a sweet treat that still powers up their health. These mini treats are a great snack for you—and your little ones.

INGREDIENTS:

1 cup gluten-free oat flour

½ cup almond flour

½ cup millet flour (or more almond flour)

4 tbsp. flax meal (or ground chia seeds)

½ tsp. baking soda

dash of cinnamon

½ cup sweetened vanilla almond milk, warm

5 tbsp. maple syrup

3 tbsp. applesauce

1 tbsp. coconut oil, warm (or canola oil)

2 tsp. apple cider vinegar

1 tsp. vanilla

¼ cup vegan chocolate chips

DIRECTIONS:

1. Preheat oven to 325°F and lightly grease a mini muffin pan or line cups with muffin liners.
2. In a bowl, whisk together all the dry ingredients.
3. In another bowl, mix together all the wet ingredients. When adding the coconut oil, make sure the wet ingredients are at room temperature to prevent the coconut oil from hardening.
4. Pour the wet ingredients over the dry and stir until consistency is smooth. Then fold in the chocolate chips.
5. Generously pour batter into 12 mini muffin cups and top with extra chocolate chips (optional).

6. Bake for about 30 minutes, or until you can slide a knife into the center and it comes out clean. Remove from oven and let cool. Then transfer muffins to a wire rack to completely cool.

7. Store in an airtight container or in plastic wrap at room temperature for a few days, or refrigerate for a week. Can also be stored in the freezer for a few months.

8. Brownie muffin option: Add 2 tbsp. cocoa powder to the dry ingredient bowl plus 2 tbsp. maple syrup to the wet ingredient bowl.

9. Enjoy a healthy and nutritious muffin for a light breakfast or as a snack!

Conclusion

START YOUR REVOLUTION TODAY!

CHANGE IS POSSIBLE. CHANGE IS continuous. Change has to start somewhere—and I'm hoping that reading this book has inspired you to start here, now, and today. Because it is possible to re-invent yourself, improve the quality of your life, and feel incredible every single day.

I have seen it time and time again. No matter who you are, what your health profile is right now, or what your habits are, if you want to change, you can. You just have to decide to do it and know you can do it. What is "it"? It's eating plants. If you've read this far, you've already read the science. You've read the success stories. You've seen the recipes—and hopefully been tantalized.

Now I want you to go from wanting to doing. From dreaming to achieving. From wondering what it would be like to succeed to actually beginning the process of success.

I wrote this book because I know for a fact that eating plants will revolutionize your experience in this world and make it more joyous, more meaningful, more vital. So try it. Try it for a meal, for a day . . . and another day . . . and another. Go the full 22 days. See what it feels like to succeed.

Give yourself the change—and the chance—that you deserve.

APPENDIX

GLOSSARY OF KEY VITAMINS

VITAMIN A: Vitamin A gives you healthy eyes, teeth, bones, and skin. You can find it in dark leafy vegetables, sweet potatoes, carrots, red peppers, cantaloupe and dark orange fruits.

VITAMIN B$_2$: Vitamin B$_2$, also known as riboflavin, is needed for energy metabolism, normal vision and skin health. It is found in green leafy vegetables and whole grains.

VITAMIN B$_{12}$: Vitamin B$_{12}$ is needed for making new cells and important for nerve function. It is not commonly found in plant-based foods.

VITAMIN C: Vitamin C (ascorbic acid) is for healing wounds, healthy teeth and gums, protein metabolism, immune health and iron absorption. Go for Brussels sprouts, cabbage, potatoes, cauliflower, peppers, citrus fruits, kiwi fruit, mangoes and strawberries.

VITAMIN D: Vitamin D is important for healthy bones and teeth. If you get 15 minutes of sunlight each day, your body can produce vitamin D! Either way, eating mushrooms will help get you in the D. Keep in mind that your body also needs vitamin D in order to absorb calcium. If there's any doubt as to whether you're getting enough vitamin D on a daily basis, talk to your physician and/or look for a plant-based supplement.

VITAMIN E: Vitamin E helps your body make red blood cells. Eat plenty of green leafy vegetables, whole grains, avocado, broccoli, asparagus, papaya, seeds, and nuts.

VITAMIN K: Vitamin K is important for blood clotting, and it helps your body use calcium to strengthen your bones. You can find it in cabbage, cauliflower, and all your green vegetables.

BIOTIN: Biotin, also known as vitamin H, is necessary in order for your body to metabolize macronutrients to give you energy. It is also useful for strengthening hair and nails. You can find it in chocolate, grains, legumes, and nuts.[71]

FOLATE: Folate is needed for the production of DNA, and is especially important for pregnant women. Eat plenty of asparagus, broccoli, beets, lentils, oranges.

NIACIN: Niacin (vitamin B_3) supports healthy skin and nerves. Choose green leafy vegetables, avocado, legumes, nuts, and potatoes.

PANTOTHENIC ACID: Pantothenic acid helps you metabolize the food you eat, including your sources of pantothenic acid: avocado, broccoli, legumes, lentils, mushrooms.

PYRIDOXINE: Pyridoxine (vitamin B_6) maintains brain function, so to keep thinking clearly, eat bananas, legumes, nuts, and whole grains.

THIAMINE: Thiamine (vitamin B_1) helps your body turn carbohydrates into usable energy. Find it in legumes, nuts, seeds, and peas.

---

[71] http://umshoreregional.org/health/medical/altmed/supplement/vitamin-h-biotin, accessed August 18, 2014.

ACKNOWLEDGMENTS

"This is a wonderful day. I've never seen this one before."
—*Maya Angelou*

I am full of gratitude!! There are people for whom without I would not be me. For this, I am eternally grateful and would like to give special thanks. To my mother, for teaching me the importance of hard work and perseverance. My brother, Alfredo, for his ability to manifest his dreams. My sister, Jennifer, for her love, kindness, positivity and dedication. My grandmother Mima for showing me you can be funny, brave, kind and adventurous all before noon and my uncle Paul for creating the spark that would eventually fuel my dreams.

A very special thank-you to Jay and BB for a friendship like no other and for their love and trust in everything we do. Thank you!!

This project has been a collaboration that leaves me humbled and grateful.

A heartfelt thank-you to my wonderful friend and publisher, Raymond Garcia, for believing and trusting in my abilities and for trying the 22 Day Challenge before it was even a concept for a book (he lost sixty-five pounds as a result of it).

Very special thanks to Sandra Bark for her incredibly curious mind and her help turning thoughts into words. Thank you! A heartfelt thank-you to Jen Schuster for smiling while pushing, dotting and crossing (oh, and on top of it all, removing some extra exclamation marks). Thank you to Arlene, Ben, Nicole and Sydney for their beautiful designs and kindness. A special thanks to my good friend Marc Leffin for his friendship and trust. And a very special thank-you to our team at

22 Days Nutrition for their hard work, dedication and belief that we can make a difference.

Special appreciation to the incredibly gifted doctors who inspire the best in me and whose brilliant work empowers millions around the world to achieve optimum wellness: Dr. Dean Ornish, Dr. Neal Barnard, Dr. Caldwell Esselstyn and Dr. Colin Campbell.

Lastly, a heartfelt thanks to my best friends, Marilyn, Marco Jr., Mateo and Maximo, for filling my life with love and for their willingness to join me on this journey. I love you with all my heart!!

INDEX